A Part of Ourselves

Also available from A. & A. Farmar

Miscarriage and Stillbirth—A Human Insight Karina Colgan

Children's Last Days Anna Farmar

Home: An Anthology of Modern Irish Writing Edited by Siobhán Parkinson

A Part of Ourselves

*Laments for Lives
that Ended too Soon*

Edited by

Siobhán Parkinson

A. & A. Farmar

British Library Cataloguing in Publication Data
A CIP catalogue record for this book is available from the British Library

Cover photographs by Derek Speirs
Cover and text design by Dunbar Design
Typesetting by A. & A. Farmar
Printed by βetaprint

ISBN 1 899047 34 4

A. & A. Farmar
Beech House
78 Ranelagh Village
Dublin 6
Ireland

If James did nothing else, he taught me how very lucky I am to have two healthy children, how miraculous and beautiful and perfect they are. And I go on realising that with an intensity which doesn't seem to dim . . . it is a gift to have been shown that and to know it so surely.

Mary Butler *Born to Die*

'None of us would have chosen that our child would die, but there was something honourable about it, there was a certain pride at the end of it. We did what we could and we did it to the best of our ability and we have no regrets. We are sad and we'll always have the sadness, but we'll also have our pride . . .'

'He's safe now. It was a privilege, we looked after him from the cradle to the grave. Death isn't the most terrible thing that can happen to anyone. If you have loved and experienced love, you have everything.'

Parents quoted in *Children's Last Days* by Anna Farmar

CONTENTS

PART 1

A Star Plummeted to Earth

PART 2

One Piece Missing

PART 3

A Windblown Spark

PART 4

That Was My First Death

PART 5

An Inextricable Love

PART 6

The Year the Spring Didn't Come

The Irish Sudden Infant Death Association

Twenty-one years ago a letter from a newly-bereaved mother whose baby had died suddenly and unexpectedly appeared in *The Irish Times*. In response, bereaved parents, professionals and friends came together to support each other in their common loss and to understand how their children died and so the Irish Sudden Infant Death Association (ISIDA) was formed.

As ISIDA heads into the new millennium, it continues to provide support to families bereaved by sudden infant death, to educate professionals, the media and the public, and to fund or support research into how a healthy child dies.

Over the past twenty-one years more than 2,300 children have died suddenly and inexplicably in Ireland because of Sudden Infant Death Syndrome (Cot Death) and sadly each week this tragedy continues to strike. Innumerable parents, siblings, relatives, friends, health care workers and other professionals each day experience a depth of emotion around the death of these children.

Today, because of ISIDA's National Sudden Infant Death Register, established in 1992, ISIDA can acknowledge every family whose lives are touched by grieving for the sudden, unexpected death of their child. Yet thousands of others unknown, unacknowledged and unsupported grieve the death of a child, brother, sister, niece, nephew, or mourn where the birth of a child has eluded them. Each individual's experience is unique, yet there is a common bond of grieving the loss of a child and the loss of what might have been. It is this spirit of reaching out that ISIDA has sought to harness in publishing this anthology. *A Part of Ourselves* is what these children who are not with us *are*, and the writings in this book reflect this.

Michéal Ó Doibhilin
Chairman
ISIDA
October 1997

Introduction

SIOBHÁN PARKINSON

I

This is a book for those who mourn the loss of a child. Of all griefs, this is surely the most profound, for it seems to fly in the face of nature that a parent should bury a child. As one parent put it in Anna Farmar's *Children's Last Days*: 'Nothing prepares you for the loss of a child. I had lost my parents, but a child . . .' We explain death to small children as what happens when a person's body gets old and tired and worn out, but how can we explain it, even to ourselves, when the one who dies is on the threshold of life—a young woman murdered by wicked men, a young man killed in a fire or a motor accident, a child victim of leukaemia, a 'cot death', a stillbirth, a miscarriage? Such deaths all have causes, known or unknown, but they appear to have no reasons.

It is human nature to look for reasons. Some of us blame the evil that we identify as having robbed us of our children—Sellafield, war, God, some pervert or criminal, medical incompetence, toxic chemicals, or our own negligence or carelessness or sheer undeserving nature. We were not worthy, we may believe, to be the parent of such a child.

In time, if we are lucky and reasonably balanced and extremely well supported, we come to relinquish our hatred for whatever it was we blame for our loss, but we do not relinquish our grief:

> Parents do not 'get over' the death of their child . . . Although the intensity of the mourning eventually diminishes with time, bereaved parents have continually to work at accepting and living with loss.
>
> *Children's Last Days*

We experience the death of a child as a uniquely devastating bereavement. Not only have we suffered a great loss, but we feel that we have failed our children. As parents we dedicate our lives to the children who are entrusted to us, and we have, we feel, dishonoured that most precious trust. We have failed to save our children from the ultimate separation, we have abandoned them to terror, we have let them go into that good night, that final darkness, where they are beyond our protection and our care.

Modern western parents are perhaps uniquely unprepared for the shock of the death of a child and may be uniquely unsupported in that loss, in comparison with parents of previous generations and other parts of the world. A combination of modern advances in immunology, obstetrics and paediatrics and the widespread practice of contraception has given the modern parent an illusion of control over family life that was unknown fifty or even twenty years ago. Accidents have always happened, but the childhood diseases that wiped out thousands of children even well into this century have been largely eradicated and childbirth is no longer quite the risky business it was. These are, of course, welcome developments, but they have led to a situation where the death of a child in western society is so unusual as to be almost taboo. The combination of a natural recoiling from so gloomy a prospect and the sheer low statistical probability of its happening to any particular individual or family has made the topic of child death one that people find particularly difficult to contemplate, much less discuss. This is no doubt a healthy strategy of self-protection among the unbereaved, but it can make the burden of the bereaved family even more difficult. Even a generation or two ago, most families had experienced some sort of child loss; but today's bereaved parent is more alone than ever.

And yet it is everywhere. When I was looking for material for this book, it seemed I couldn't open a book in a shop or a library or a friend's house but the theme of child loss came leaping out at me from the pages. It is everywhere and at the same time it is taboo, unspoken, unacknowledged.

This book, a collection of laments by Irish writers for lives that ended too soon, seeks to give voice to that largely unarticulated and unacknowledged grief. It brings a message to families that are bereaved in this way, and the message is not one of hope or one of consolation or one of damage-limitation. The message is very simple: you are not alone. However unacknowledged your grief may seem to be by the culture at large, it is a grief that is shared by other women and men, mothers and fathers, brothers and sisters, grandparents and friends. A grief shared is not a grief halved: it is simply a grief shared. But a grief shared is surely an experience of human communication that goes beyond the normal experience of social intercourse or of literary achievement.

However we grieve, however we deal with our loss, a universal of mourning a child seems to be the feeling that whatever happens, this child remains for ever 'a part of ourselves'—hence the title of this book, taken from Peter Fallon's fine poem on the death of his infant son. There is an almost eerie echo of that phrase in the words of another parent: 'He is part of my life and always will be.' (Mary Butler *Born to Die*). To all those who mourn the passing of a part of themselves this book is dedicated.

II

All the poems and prose pieces in this book were written by poets and authors who are Irish by birth or association. Many of the contributions are by well-known poets and writers, but some are by 'ordinary' parents and friends. Most of the contributions were published previously, but some are new. Most are by people who have themselves experienced child bereavement or whose family has had such an experience, and some are by people who have not but who recognise the loss of a child as a parent's greatest fear and who have written in empathy with friends or fictional characters who have had that experience. Where the author of a piece volunteered personal information about the cirumstances of writing the piece, this has been included.

The book consists of six sections, each named from a poem or prose piece in the section. The first two sections, 'A Star Plummeted to Earth' and 'One Piece Missing', comprise poetry and prose respectively about the loss of a child by a parent or from the perspective of a parent. The next section, 'A Windblown Spark', is about the loss of a child from the perspective of an outsider, a family member, friend or simply someone who has been moved to empathy by the idea of child death. 'That Was my First Death' is about the loss of a sibling in childhood or early adulthood.

Sections 5 and 6 push out the theme of child loss into other areas: 'An Inextricable Love' is about the loss of a child not involving death—for example by giving up for adoption or by emigration; and 'The Year the Spring Didn't Come' consists of contributions on childlessness—the loss, in a sense, of what never was, a most particular grief.

Acknowledgements

The editor thanks the following people for their support and for suggestions for poems and extracts to include in the book: Roger Bennett, Mairéad Carew, Anna Farmar, Mary Jennings, Phil MacCarthy, Niall McMonagle.

The authors have generously donated the royalties from the sale of this volume to the Irish Sudden Infant Death Association. The Association and A. & A. Farmar thank the authors and authors' heirs for their generosity in this regard.

PUBLICATION DETAILS

Eavan Boland, 'Child of Our Time', 'The Famine Road' and 'The Pomegranate' from *Collected Poems*, published by Carcanet Press, 1995

Rory Brennan, 'A Child That Didn't Live', from *The Old in Rapallo* (1996), published by Salmon Publishing Ltd, The Cliffs of Moher, Co. Clare

Evelyn Conlon, 'Birth Certificates', from *Taking Scarlet as a Real Colour* (1993), published by Blackstaff Press

Peter Cunningham, extract from *Who Trespass Against Us* (1994), published by Arrow Books

John F Deane, 'Gillin na Leanbh', from *High Sacrifice* (1991), published by Dolmen

Seamus Deane, extract from *Reading in the Dark* (1996), published by Jonathan Cape

Alison Dye, extract from *Memories of Snow* (1995), published by Sceptre

Peter Fallon, 'A Part of Ourselves', from *Eye to Eye* (1992), by kind permission of the author and The Gallery Press

Hugo Hamilton, extract from *The Love Test* (1995), published by Faber and Faber

Jack Hanna, for 'Lilies and Daffodils' by Davoren Hanna, from *The Friendship Tree, The Life and Poetry of Davoren Hanna*, published by New Island Books

Kerrie Hardie, 'A Childless Woman', from *A Furious Place* (1996), by kind permission of the author and The Gallery Press

Michael Hartnett, 'The Night Before Patricia's Funeral' and 'For Edward Hartnett', from *Selected Poems* (1970), published by Zozimus/New Writers Press

Seamus Heaney, 'Limbo' from *Wintering Out* (1972), 'Elegy for a Stillborn Child', from *Door Into the Dark* (1969), 'Mid-Term Break', from *Death of a Naturalist* (1966), all published by Faber and Faber

Winifred Letts, 'Easter Snow', published in *Songs of Leinster*

Catherine Phil MacCarthy, 'Nativity' and 'Birth Mother' from *This Hour of the Tide* (1994), Salmon Publishing Ltd, The Cliffs of Moher, Co. Clare

Deirdre Madden, extract from *Birds of the Innocent Wood* (1988), published by Faber and Faber

Alf McCreary, extract from *Gordon Wilson: An Ordinary Hero*, published by Harper Collins

Patsy McGarry, 'Not Just "The Baby"', from 'An Irishman's Diary' by kind permission of *The Irish Times*

John MacKenna, 'Absent Child', from *A Year of Our Lives* (1996), published by Picador

Paula Meehan, 'Elegy for a Child' and 'Child Burial', from *The Man Who Was Marked by Winter* (1991), by kind permission of The Gallery Press

Kuno Meyer, 'The Mothers' Lament at the Slaughter of the Innocents', from *Ancient Irish Poetry*, published by Constable

Mary Morrissy, extract from *Mother of Pearl* (1996), published by Jonathan Cape

Nuala Ní Dhomhnaill, 'Breith Anabaí Thar Lear/Miscarriage Abroad', from *Selected Poems* (1988), published by Raven Arts

Eilís Ní Dhuibhne, 'The Garden of Eden' from *Eating Women is not Recommended*, published by Attic Press

Mairtín Ó Cadhain, 'The Year 1912', from *The Road to Bright City*, translated by Eoghan Ó Tuairisc, published by Poolbeg

Mary O'Donnell, 'Antartica' and 'Cot Death', from *Reading the Sunflowers in September* (1990), published by Salmon Publishing Ltd, The Cliffs of Moher, Co. Clare, extract from *The Light-Makers*, published by Poolbeg

Bernard O'Donoghue, 'Áine', from *Gunpowder* (1995), published by Chatto and Windus

Dennis O'Driscoll, 'Stillborn' originally published in *Hidden Extras*, published by Anvil Press, London, Dedalus Press, Dublin

Nuala O'Faoláin, extract from *Are You Somebody?*, published by New Island Books

Sheila O'Hagan, 'Elegy for Mark' from *The Troubled House* (1994), published by Salmon Publishing Ltd, The Cliffs of Moher, Co. Clare

Cathal Ó Searcaigh, 'Nuair ba Ghnách liom Luí le mo Thuismitheoirí', from *Na Buachaillí Bána* (1996), published by Cló Iar-Chonnachta Teo.

Derry O'Sullivan, 'Marbhghin 1943: Glaoch ar Liombó/Stillborn 1943: A Call to Limbo', from *Irish Poetry Now* (1993), published by Wolfhound Press; 'Cot Death' translated from Gaelic by the author, published by First Impressions, Paris 1987.

Elizabeth Peavoy, 'The Day We Drove Down La Nicolière' was published in *Cork Review 16*.

Janet Shepperson, 'The Aphrodite Stone' and 'Childless', from *The Aphrodite Stone*, published by Salmon Publishing Ltd, The Cliffs of Moher, Co. Clare

James Simmons, 'Elegy for a Dead-Born Child', from *Mainstream*, published by Salmon Publishing Ltd, The Cliffs of Moher, Co. Clare

Jason Sommer, 'Not when you call them do the pictures come', from *Lifting the Stone* (1991), published by Forest Books, Specialists in International Literature, ISBN 0 948259 94 9, price £6.95

PART 1

A Star Plummeted to Earth

Elegy for a Child

PAULA MEEHAN

It is not that the spring brings
you back. Birds riotous about
the house, fledglings learn to fly.

Nor that coming on petals drifted in the orchard
is like opening your door, a draught of pastel,
a magpie hoard of useless bright.

Clouds move over the river
under the sun—a cotton sheet shook out.
The pines bring me news
from deeper in the woods:
the rain will come sing on the roof soon.

It is not the day's work in the garden,
the seedlings neatly leafmould mulched in lines.
Not the woodpile trim bespeaking good husbandry,
conjuring up the might-have-been.

It is not the anarchic stream
in a stone-sucking dash past the crane's haunt, fickle,
sky mirror now, now shattered bauble,

nor the knowledge of planets in proper order,
their passage through my fourth house
fixed before I was born.
It is not that the night you died
a star plummeted to earth.
It is not that I watched it fall.

It is not that I was your mother,
nor the rooted deep down loss,
that has brought me this moment
to sit by the window and weep.

You were but a small bird balanced
within me
ready for flight.

Child Burial

PAULA MEEHAN

Your coffin looked unreal,
fancy as a wedding cake.

I chose your grave clothes with care,
your favourite stripey shirt,

your blue cotton trousers.
They smelt of woodsmoke, of October,

your own smell there too.
I chose a gansy of handspun wool,

warm and fleecy for you. It is
so cold down in the dark.

No light can reach you and teach you
the paths of wild birds,

the names of the flowers,
the fishes, the creatures.

Ignorant you must remain
of the sun and its work,

my lamb, my calf, my eaglet,
my cub, my kid, my nestling,

my suckling, my colt. I would spin
time back, take you again

within my womb, your amniotic lair,
and further spin you back

through nine waxing months
to the split seeding moment

you chose to be made flesh,
word within me.

I'd cancel the love feast
the hot night of your making.

I would travel alone
to a quiet mossy place,

you would spill from me into the earth
drop by bright red drop.

Breith Anabaí Thar Lear

NUALA NÍ DHOMHNAILL

Luaimnigh do shíol i mo bhroinn,
d'fháiltíos roimh do bhreith.
Dúrt go dtógfainn go cáiréiseach thú
de réir gnása mo nuamhuintire.

An leabhar beannaithe faoi do philiúr
arán is snáthaid i do chliabhán,
léine t'athar anuas ort
is ag do cheann an scuab urláir.

Bhí mo shonas
ag cur thar maoil
go dtí sa deireadh
gur bhris na bainc
is sceith
frog deich seachtainí;
ní mar a shíltear a bhí.

Is anois le teacht na Márta
is an bhreith a bhí
le breith i ndán duit
cuireann ribíní bána na taoide
do bhindealáin i gcuimhne dom,
tointe fada na hóinsí.

Is ní raghad
ag féachaint linbh
nuabheirthe mo dhlúthcharad
ar eagla mo shúil mhillteach
do luí air le formad.

Miscarriage Abroad

NUALA NÍ DHOMHNAILL

Translated by Michael Hartnett

I had a miscarriage, and about the time the child would have been due I found myself thinking about it. Everyone I spoke to about it said I was mad, and should have got over it by now—hence, 'tointe fada na hóinsí'—even the froth of the sea reminded me of the snagged thread of life which had broken. The poem was a fundamental part of the grieving process.

You, embryo, moved in me—
I welcomed your emerging
I said I'd rear you carefully
in the manner of my new people—

under your pillow the holy book,
in your cot, bread and a needle:
your father's shirt as an eiderdown
at your head a brush for sweeping.

I was brimming
with happiness
until the dykes broke
and out was swept
a ten-weeks frog—
'the best-laid schemes . . .'

And now it's March
your birthday that never was—
and white ribbons of tide
remind me of baby-clothes,
an imbecile's tangled threads.

And I will not go to see
my best friend's new born child
because of the jealousy
that stares from my evil eye.

Nativity

CATHERINE PHIL MacCARTHY

We kiss and when you
leave for work
I notice the figures

you made of modelling clay
blue, green, yellow
all over our house

the night before,
lovingly moulding shapes
to stave off grief

your hands worried flesh,
all the care you took
taunting me with loss.

The Aphrodite Stone

JANET SHEPPERSON

The stone is what I've salvaged
from winter-bruised Akamas, the limestone cliffs
that curl into caves and grottoes, crumble
into a wave-locked Burren where thistle and thorn
nuzzle apart the vertebrae of rock
and the tide is all the music
of pebbles grinding churning abrading hammering
holes in each other.

The stone is a sculpture
by Henry Moore, with a gap hollowed out
where the heart and guts should be.

The stone is a woman
crouched on the edge of the bed. She cradles
her breasts that still hang heavy, blindly seeking
tiny mouths to suck, refusing to be
comforted, refusing to know
that the child was never a child but a clot of blood
ebbing out of her
leaving a cavity
for the wind to whistle through.

The stone is a souvenir
from Aphrodite's birthplace from the rock
where she perched like a mermaid posing for the tourists
till her honey-coloured flesh faded to grey
weathered fractured fissured pock-marked pocketed

into holes and then worn smooth
by the undertow,
abandoned
above high water mark.

The stone says: Hold me
in the hollow of your hand.

The Night Before Patricia's Funeral

MICHAEL HARTNETT

the night before Patricia's funeral in 1951,
I stayed up late talking to my father.

how goes the night, boy?
   the moon is down:
   dark is the town
   in this nightfall.
how goes the night, boy?
   soon is her funeral,
   her small white burial.
she was my threeyears child,
her honey hair, her eyes
small ovals of thrush-eggs.
how goes the night, boy?
   it is late: lace
   at the window
   blows back in the wind.
how goes the night, boy?
   —Oh, my poor white fawn!
how goes the night, boy?
   it is dawn.

Cot Death

MARY O'DONNELL

This poem emerged from combined impulses: my interest in Irish folklore and a contemporary consideration of the question of parental guilt. W. B. Yeats' poem 'The Stolen Child' was somewhere at the back of my mind, too, its sinister yet seductive atmosphere, its note of warning regarding life's melancholic undertow . . .

When I turned her over,
what I saw was a changeling's mask,
mauve and mottled, like old lilac,
her lips purpled shut.

No flutter from her eyelashes
that always quivered
like down on a young bird,
and I knew how her nostrils,

the pink-edged membranes,
were inhabited by death,
how the sculpting of her ears
had nothing now to do with sound.

Since then, I am haunted awake,
a wailing behind my temples,
and I grit my teeth each time
I see dolls in snug shop windows,

their glassy eyes accusatory,
knowing them to be corpses
subpoenaed for a public enquiry
into some woman's unmotherly neglect.
I will always wonder if

those matrons who shun me lest
I conjure a changeling to their doors,
are not correct, I will wonder

if I invoked some blood-curdling sprite
to suffocate the child before she
suffocated me. And wondering,
I am haunted, I am unstill,

my days waxing murderously.

Haikus

MAIRÉAD CAREW

My baby daughter, Órfhlaith McDonald, died on 2 January 1996 in a cot death, aged seven months.

In an angel's arms
You left in darkness
in the gap between heartbeats
in an angel's arms

Loss
Our tears blend with rain
tinning a cadence of loss
on galvanised roofs

Snowflake
A snowflake melting
on a January day
to remember you

Summer leaves
I hear her soft voice
sing in a whisper of wind
rustling summer leaves

When the cocoon breaks
When the cocoon breaks
the butterfly emerges
flapping its new wings

Prayer
I will kneel and pray
for a warm nest of silence
to envelop you

To Sophie

ROZ COWMAN

This is the first poem I ever wrote. My baby daughter, Sophie, died in May 1973. I wrote this poem around October 1974, when I was still crippled by losing her. I wrote, not to 'write a poem' but to try to make clear to myself what had happened to us both—the feeling that I had died with her, but was still alive enough to feel pain.

Host and companion to your unborn days,
beloved mentor in your new-found
world; and when my eyes
were dazzled by the blaze of love,
you left, and leaving
took my soul with you.

Stillborn

DENNIS O'DRISCOLL

My poem, 'Stillborn', arose not from personal experience but from deep empathy. When the wife of a good friend and office colleague had borne her second stillborn baby (each after a full nine-month term), there seemed no words left that would comfort or console. The words that did come—and which I hesitantly placed in the heartbroken parents' mouths—formed both a nursery rhyme and a lament, a lullaby and an elegy.

what we are lamenting
is what has not been
and what will not have seen
this mild May morning

what we are lamenting
is unsuckled air
and what was brought to bear
this mild May morning

what we are lamenting
is the blood and puppy fat, our child,
that has not laughed or cried
this mild May morning

what we are lamenting
is the life we crave
snatched from the cradle to the grave
this mild May morning

Elegy for a Deadborn Child

JAMES SIMMONS

Up stepped the cabin boy and bravely out spoke he.
He said to the captain, 'What will you give me,
if I will swim alongside the Spanish enemy
and sink her in the lowlands lowlands low,
sink her in the lowland sea?'
The Golden Vanity

1
A brief addition to the family
shown and withdrawn in the longest moment of my life.

all our concern was how to help my wife
endure and survive bearing a dead baby,
all that intrusion, bruising and abuse.

An Indian doctor told us the law said
she must be satisfied the child was dead
before the mother could be treated, induce
labour and get that clot of blood excreted,
remove what now we waited for with dread.

Most of the day we waited.

2
This morning was a holiday. After we woke
we made love. Then suddenly the waters broke.
There should be absolutely no connection
all the doctors insisted. However you thrust
up the vagina the hardest erection
it never troubles the small life held in trust.
The waters broke. The mildest irritation
of wet sheets, and slowly the implication.

The ignorant husband had to be told no embryo
survives the drying up of the amniotic sea.
She gradually brought it home to me.
I had plans for the morning that I must forego.

3
Different doctors on duty had different views,
the nurses made sour faces. It was easy to lose
track. Experts don't always want to say
what they know. Patients are at their mercy.
A corpse in the womb is suddenly dangerous.
The mother is naturally loath to make a fuss,

pretty and clean in her cotton shift, her mind
grinding to grasp problems, her nerves strained.

Then they came in to inject her. They wheeled her away,
me following, then banished, then restored. I had no say.

'You're doing great, dear,' said a coarse
assistant. 'Push down, hard, to your arse.
Lovely. Push down again, like a hard shit.'

So gods are born. She was glad to be rid of it.

That mind, that body tests the hospital,
nurses and surgeons. In her, nature is ill.
Even the architect, the administration
bear down on her, their skill and limitation.
Nature is fighting nature, their illness fights
her illness. The woman bleeds under the lights.

4
Four inches long, on folded cotton wool
whatever it was lay,
fleshy, like a pork fillet on a butcher's tray,

skin that transparent
and he pointedly wasn't looking at you,
exact and remote, a small bronze statue.

Closer, his big head was shapely, one arm
folded across a wren-bone chest,
the tiny hands poised, halted
in some activity. No harm
had come to the long fingers, but he was dead.
The little cabin boy had done his best.

We were learning him, like our other little one.
He was like him in miniature, and Ben is small enough.
A brother then, somebody worth mourning.
Mother and father released at last from the rough
mismanagement of hospitals, learning
a sense of loss and reward, to love their son.

5
As we looked and touched
questions were put to us
by nurse and doctor,
how to dispose of this?

To us, tragic and rarely:
to them, unfortunate but daily.
Us, shocked, inclined to hurt,
but resentment was silly.

We could take the thing home,
make of our garden
a private graveyard
with a single headstone,

or make his bed under the roses
or store his ashes in vases,
or leave him lying
where the admin disposes.

Not home surely!
Our bad dog, Charlie,
would smell out meat
and resurrect him early.

We were hard put to decide,
until formaldehyde
the preserver was suggested.
That left us goggle-eyed.

Let the administrator
dispose of the little creature
in whatever usual way,
dustbin or incinerator.

Only in heart and memory
let him survive. Bury him
silent, invisible,
within us, without ceremony.

6
I always hated magic.
I lost Jesus for that.
Let happen whatever happens,
let the dead lie
stinking of death and life,
finished, flat.
Let all who knew him
exercise memory.

To be born dead
is to be wondered at,
and I wonder.
No one is going to cry.
The wake
will be very private.

7
Released at last
from that stark theatre,
the steel bowls and blood,
the bleak unhomeliness,
a warehouse, an empty supermarket,

I wheeled you back
to the private bedroom,
its high windows brimming
with green blue sky
of gorgeous evening
after the long day.

We could lie together,
the bruised, bereaved mother,
and her tired lover, semi-conscious
of a pelmet of wispy clouds
being drawn across
the glowing shell of moon.

We were part of the long hot summer of '89
again, exiled in Belfast's Royal Hospital
from our new home by the sea, everything
bad happening and never happier.

My mother
was half a mile away,
down in the city,

slowly and reluctantly
loosing her tough old
hold on life.

8

I drifted back in history,
living another blazing summer,
relished in Donegal
with a different cast
of loved ones, lost now,

one who went off
to England—no bother—
for an abortion
and returned smiling.
She said, 'The day after
we walked down to the station,
three girls with our wee cases.
It was a holiday.'

9

Janice, you've heard me calling Ben
Charlie, the dog's name, when
I was tired. And Anna, it's well known,
I call by the names of children
with children of their own,
so separate lives get mixed and blend,
Ben and our dead embryo, Helen and Anna.
I like that mystic feel. I cry 'Hosannah'
for birth, for parenthood. Can you let me say,
'Anna is Rachael is Helen is Penelope?'
And I've called you by the names of previous
wives, shuffling my past and duplicating lives.
I stand by this: my mother did the same.
Don't think these quirks insulting or inane,

I was my father, Stewart, to her or my nephew,
Michael, males who at different times she knew
by the one tie of her love, for eternity,
petering out now in Ward 23
in stray smiles, as her mind holds or slips.
I consult my watch, and kiss her withered lips.
Love is confusing, in the surge and relapse
we all fill gaps in other lives and leave gaps
to be filled. Leave my mistakes uncorrected
In confusion the lost lovers are less neglected.
And if you start calling me Don Paul after
your Scottish lover, promise each other laughter
not hurt, embarrassment or accusation.
Bow to the good times. Honour collaboration.

10
Your eyes closed. When your breath was regular
I walked alone down long bright corridors,
unlocked our battered Peugeot and drove home.
Somewhere along the way I stopped involuntarily,
maybe exhausted, and slumped over the wheel,
embracing an old friend who always starts
in the morning and takes us where we have to go.
The son and sister I am driving to
will wait. I sensed above me, above the city
up in the evening sky, something going home,
like one of the lighter planes you see lose height,
down, out of sight, to the harbour. That was my own
son, a failed impulse from the teeming earth
returned, too little, and too lately known.

His mates they dragged him up, and on the deck he died.
They sewed him in his hammock that was so fair and wide,
then they lowered him overboard and he's drifting with the
tide,
drifting in the lowlands, lowlands low,
drifting in the lowland sea.

The Day We Drove Down La Nicolière

Elizabeth Peavoy

Our third child, Eliza, died in Mauritius where the family was living. She was fourteen months old when she died, on 30th June 1979, and was buried in St Pierre cemetery. Her name is inscribed on our family headstone in Navan, Co. Meath.

After you died I had nothing but regret
a bunch of graveyard roses no use
to anyone least of all you. Yet I remember
the day we drove down la Nicolière
and you too sick for anything least of all
driving down a mountain pass. I had never
seen anything that sick before as you dear
and didn't know quite what to fear
yet I feared and fought holding your will
to live in mine for you now I alone
must hold a bunch of Christmas Roses

hard to believe in that existence beyond
graveyards, but you had a mouth pink peony
cheeks a nose and eyes for laughter
and pearly hands for reaching out and grasping
the silver strings from heaven pulling you.
Why the hurt so great to have the child
one loves depart for what they say
becomes a better life leaving her spoon
bowl there with saccharine poetry to scar
and simplify our hearts. Gone with white dress
my dear and your almost smiles.

The Mothers' Lament at the
Slaughter of the Innocents

KUNO MEYER

(Translated from the 11th-century Irish)

Then, as the executioner plucked her son from her
　　breast, one of the women said:

Why do you tear from me my darling son,
The fruit of my womb?
It was I who bore him,
My breast he drank,
My womb carried him about,
My vitals he sucked,
My heart he filled.
He was my life,
'Tis death to have him taken from me.
My strength has ebbed,
My speech is silenced,
My eyes are blinded.

Then another woman said:

It is my son you take from me.
I did not do the evil,
But kill me—me!
Kill not my son!
My breasts are sapless,
My eyes are wet,
My hands shake,
My poor body totters.
My husband has no son,
And I no strength.
My life is like death.

O my own son, O God!
My youth without reward,
My birthless sicknesses
Without requital until Doom.
My breasts are silent,
My heart is wrung.

Then said another woman:

Ye are seeking to kill one,
Ye are killing many.
Infants ye slay,
The fathers ye wound,
The mothers ye kill.
Hell with your deed is full,
Heaven is shut,
Ye have spilt the blood of guiltless innocents.

And yet another woman said:

O Christ, come to me!
With my son take my soul quickly!
O great Mary, Mother of God's Son,
What shall I do without my son?
For Thy Son my spirit and sense are killed.
I am become a crazy woman for my son.
After the piteous slaughter
My heart is a clot of blood
From this day till Doom.

Easter Snow

WINIFRED LETTS

My jewel of the world, she sleeps so fast,
She will not hear you, Spring wind, if you blow;
So let you shake the blossoms of the thorn
Till her bed is hidden deep in Easter snow.

Bright jewel of my heart, she sleeps at last,
O kind Earth, wrap her round in your brown shawl.
Sing soft to her and rock her in your arms
So she'll not be lonesome after me at all.

I hear the childher laugh as they run past,
They see their mother watching at the door;
It's long I'll wait beside the lonely hearth,
For there's sorra child of mine will cross the floor.

O thorn trees round her grave, now let you cast
Your snow upon the place she takes her rest.
The while I stay and cheat my heart with dreams
That I'm holding her again upon my breast.

A Part of Ourselves

PETER FALLON

in memory of John Fallon
born 7 December died 8 December 1990

Forewarned but not forearmed—
no, not for this.
A word first whispered months ago
and longed for longer tripped on the tongue,
a stammer, now a broken promise.

Averted eyes. Uncertain talk
of a certain strange condition.
The scanned screen slips out of focus,
a lunar scene, granite shapes, shifting.
We bent beneath the weight of attrition

knowing it might have been worse.

       *

We were visited.
Now the minutes are grief
or grief postponed—not to remember
seems to betray; laughter would be sacrilege.
We will find a way to mind him as a leaf

who fell already from the family tree,
crushed. He hadn't a chance.
We pray at best for the open wound
to grow a scar.
We welcome him his deliverance.

There are things worse than death.

*

Imagine a man not wanting to live
who could. Now he lies in an oxygen tent
in the whispered kindness of nurses.
Night and day are one to him,
his without hunger, just bewilderment

and quiet uncomplaining. Brightly lit.
He seems to breathe another air.
There's a photograph in *The Best of* LIFE:
A summary execution, Budapest, October 1956.
He flinched that way from the snapshot glare

of the world laid out for him.

*

So they gave her sedatives.
I sought and found the comfort of a friend.
She tendered brave communion
in the early hours
as I waited, waited, for the given end.

There are more hurts than cures.
Already we'd begun talking
the hushed courtesies of loss.
Then, at dawn, the telephone.
It seems I've been sleepwalking

since.

*

We broached the sorrow hoard
of women, tales unmentioned in their marriages,
unsaid to friends, to families.
Fellow feeling loosed their tongues
about unwanted pregnancies, abortions, miscarriages,
as his remains, a fingerful of hair,
a photograph, his cold kiss called, 'Remember me,'
and I stood with them at the lip
of graves. She cried from miles away,
'I miss my baby,' as an amputee

laments a phantom limb.

*

Time and again, for years on years,
I've thought about a corner of Loughcrew,
a three-foot plot for 'Henry Timson,
born and died September 2nd, 1899',
sheltered under ivy-overgrown yew,

and wondered how you'd walk away from burying
a child. Little I knew. Now the sound
of a cousin's prayers and Pa Grimes' spade
wheels me round and her sudden, 'We are leaving
a part of ourselves in that ground.'

The innocent part.

*

He'll die again at Christmas every year.
We felt the need grow all night
to give him a name, to assert him
as a member of our care, to say he was
alive. Oh, he lived all right,

he lived a lifetime. Now certain sounds,
sights and smells are the shibboleth
of a season. In a hospital corridor
I held him in my arms. I held him tight.
His mother and I, we held our breath—

and he held his.

Brother Job

MAEVE KELLY

My daughter Oona was killed in a road accident in March 1991. It took me a long time to be able to put pen to paper after her death. When I finally managed it, I found that addressing a series of poems to her gave me a place to put my grief. Of all that I had read, Job's lamentation was the one piece of writing that I could identify with. It is such a tremendously powerful poem about loss and grief, I don't think anyone could ever better it. I love Job's complaints because they are so honest and valid. Above all, I am grateful to him for sharing his ash heap with me.

When she was taken, scapegoated,
tethered to a stick one night,
in March, moonlit, clear skied,
Spring on the way, growthy things
nipping at winter's heels;
when from His hand a whirr of wings,
death with his mighty heart,
great beak open, sharp claws ready,
scooped the heart from our breast,

Then

Job made room for me.
He moved over on his ash heap
to share his space. Rheumy eyed,
leprous skinned, flaking
like dead moths into a thousand wings
we picked scabs together,
longed for death, moaned in unison,
claimed innocence of wrongdoing,

contended with the One,
complained of being curdled as cheese,
and swallowed our sour spit
with the fervour of wine tasters.

Like reeds in a desert
our tongues withered and blackened.
Our throats dried. The roots
of our hair shrivelled and whitened.
From our cracked mouths we counted
the myriad ways of God
his balancing of clouds,
his map of the thunderbolt's route,
his doors locking out the oceans,
his manylanterned stars.

Could our voices roar,
like the bellow of the chasms,
in the pit of the earth's core?
Could we spout flame or blow gases
to singe the rain forests,
that he should test us?

Job and I, comfortless,
comforted each other. Sweet brother
shared with me his affliction.
A gift beyond reckoning, a gem
set in platinum, richer than
the east's full complement
was our sorrowing together.

Vengeance is mine, saith the Lord.
What have we done, asks my brother Job?
What have we done? ask I.

Passing the Hall

MAEVE KELLY

Passing the hall,
I saw the blue brilliance
of a flower in a bowl
and caught again in passing
the acute memory of you
and felt comforted by a rose
placed in the same array,
perfect in its essence,
shape and scent, arrangement
of petals and the exact fall
of its leaf.

Your loss remains
the truest part of my nature,
yet a colour, luminous
as this May sky, brings me
to the abandoned element
that once quivered and arose
to take the bait of my muse.

Your mother's heart
so fixed in ice it could not
move beyond your death,
now takes me to a place
my grief made distant.
And now I learn again.
I'm certain that your life
has been preserved
to surface in the colour
of a flower, and I
at last begin to thaw.

Tree of Life

EAVAN BOLAND

A tree on a moonless night
has no sap or colour

It has no flower and no fruit.

It waits for the sun to find them—

if I cannot find you
in this dark hour
dear child

wait
for dawn
to make us clear to one another

for the sun
to inch above a world

where love
is the light
that shows again

the blossom
to the root.

PART2

One Piece Missing

One Piece Missing

ELEANOR FLEGG

See it as a jigsaw. A close-knit mosaic of parts spread wide between then and now. A jigsaw that is always the full picture and will never be completed. An ongoing puzzle unfolding day by day.

See it as a jigsaw with one piece missing. An unborn child that died so early that I know nothing about her other then the space she left behind. And around that little sadness the picture spreads before and after.

Here we are in Fife between the church spire and the village school. Beyond the garden the farmer is trailing a flock of gulls behind his plough. The stubbled fields are blond on either side of the turning earth. Stubble of corn and the green feathering of the winter crop. We wake to skies dappled pink and orange; the ground coated with a thick fur of frost. At night the gritter passes over the hill in a shower of salt and sand; orange lights whirling and flashing like a winter dragon heading over the brow of the hill towards Cupar.

Here we are, Tif and I; parents twice over and rulers of a crowded roost. In our house built by a council architect with materials off the back of the regional lorry. He was lavish with the window panes and driven to little flights of stairs all over the place. It is airy in summer, chilly in winter and filling rapidly with children and animals.

There is Vanya, on the brink of his fifth birthday. A cropped thatch of dark hair. Bottle-green eyes. The rooms are littered with drawings and a scattered frosting of toys. Our world is peopled with spacemen, pirates and monsters. Nightmares to be rescued from and meals to be negotiated with the bargaining skill of an expert trader. The days are a pattern of wild adventure.

Turlough is his baby brother. All milk and nappies and heartbreakingly beautiful smiles. Every day he unfolds like a little round bud. Opening his hands to the world. Two boys shouting in each other's faces with the joy of being brothers. Tuesday's children the pair of them. Full of grace.

The pony is Murdo. A woolly highlander. A round hairy barrel of a pony. We go bareback through the woods, Murdo and I, his black-tipped ears pricked forward with excitement and the dog going mad in the autumn leaves. He is the pony that I longed for as a child and waited twenty years for. Self-willed, stroppy and much loved; the fulfilment of a dream.

The dog is Brynn; hairy and thin. A lurcher who has never been able to shake off the sadness of something that happened him before he came to us. Part hound and part brillo-pad; nothing that we know how to do will keep him off the beds.

Aside from this is a golden cat and four black hens.

There's someone missing from my family. I have not given her a name. Who knows how long she lived inside me? A week maybe. A couple of weeks. Not longer.

We were living in the east of Scotland, north of Dundee and south of Aberdeen. A bleak and arable land of frozen fields and cattle herds. It was a miserable winter. A hopeless time as we drifted from one set of relatives to another in search of work and a place to live.

I walked the farmland on the hill above the house where we stayed. The sun skimmed the horizon and set early in the day. Our high hopes had foundered and it was hard work to keep our spirits up.

When I conceived in the midst of all of this it seemed that a breath of hope had blown in from a warmer climate. New life. A promise of new beginnings. It was early spring. She would have been born in October.

I miss her. I miss the times we never had together. I regret that I never saw her face. That I never held her in my arms. I believe, although I do not know, that she was a girl. It would have been good to have a daughter.

The pregnancy lasted for eleven weeks. Our hopes were rising.

I found work in Dundee and the bank agreed to a mortgage. One Saturday we drove on icy roads to see a house. A scruffy modern house. A big garden tangled with briars and early blue-bells. We were sat down and offered fine coffee and shortbread. A fire was burning in the grate. We bought the house. Despite the antiquated heating system and the proximity of the sewage works it felt like a place where we could live.

A couple of weeks before Easter I went into the hospital for a scan and found that my baby had died. No heartbeat. Not even a body, for she had died so early that her body had not had time to form. The pregnancy had continued without her.

My body had been lying to itself. For who knows how many weeks it had been building its hopes around a baby who was going no further. Although it was some consolation that her life was not hanging in the balance, I felt cheated. I did not know how to mourn the emptiness that she had left behind.

What had she been? A little knot of cells. An expectation. A sort of physical promise.

One thing I knew for certain. She had not been nothing. She had lived and died inside me and her death saddened me.

It was an unfamiliar sorrow. Something which had barely ex-isted had been taken from me. A life so slight that only four or five people knew of its passing. And a sadness that lingered long after.

It came in waves. For weeks, and later months, I would almost forget. Forget that she had been. Forget that she had gone. And then the sadness would take me unawares. It would come up behind me and put two cold hands over my eyes. I would be overtaken by a sense of loss so acute that it took my breath away. So surprising that it would be some time before I realised what was hurting me. The death of a child. And so, in fits and starts, I mourned her passing.

I took refuge in God. I did not understand why he had let a baby live inside me for a couple of weeks. Or why he had taken her away. But there is plenty that I don't understand about God. Sometimes the only thing that I do understand is that I need him. And that trusting a God who doesn't make sense is a lot better than being on your own.

It was Easter Sunday. The sun was pouring down upon the kitchen table and I was empty with loss.

And God answered me like he sometimes does. A roundabout sideways riddle of an answer.

I came back for you.

He came back. For a moment, the resurrection stood clear of the accretions of history and theology. He came back because he loves us. And however sad and confusing the world is, he has not left us alone in it. We have not been abandoned. He came back for us.

He came back in the way that a lover returns at the end of the movie. That sentimental, romantic, heart-wrenching moment. That joyous burst of relief! Mother and child. Father and son. Lover and beloved. Against all the odds he came back. And so we, the lost and bewildered, throw ourselves into his arms.

Maybe, if heaven is that sort of place, I will meet my child. I know that I'll recognise her. She'll be dark haired and sturdy like the rest of us. Maybe. If heaven is that sort of place.

I saw Turlough, my second son, on the ultrasound screen twelve weeks after he was conceived. I saw arms, legs, hands and feet. A round head and a pulsing heart. A little creature kicking his way around his water tank. Tossing and turning head over heels as though he were trying to convince me of the firm grip he had on life. The three of us watched him cavort across the screen. We asked Vanya what he saw.

A baby, he said, my brother.

What shall we call him?

Truck. That's a good name. Truck.

We tried to warn him that the brother might be a sister. We tried to get him to think of a girl's name. But he wasn't having any of it. Van and Truck. That was how it was going to be.

Absent Child

JOHN MACKENNA

I was babysitting one night and listening to Leonard Cohen when I recalled an accident that happened to one of my children—not a fatal accident. It set me thinking about loss and the terror of the loss of a child.

How often have I listened to this song? Hundreds of times, thousands, in the last fifteen years. I've learned and unlearned it again and now, tonight, I've got inside it and it's inside me. Working its way deeper than ever before, getting under my skin and under whatever it is that's under the skin.

Subconsciously, I must have known when I put the album on that there was something there, something that would unlock the agitation I've felt all day, something that would calm the unsettled way I've been since morning. But now that it's out, now that I've listened, now that I've finally heard, I know it goes back further than today. Of course it does. And this morning seems perfectly clear. Everything that happened then is clear, every shadow is clearly outlined. There's only black and white now. Darkness and light. Life and death. And calmness, yes calmness but not peace. Never peace. Never real peace. That's too much to ask for. Peace is something far beyond my expectations, beyond hope.

'Love is like smoke, beyond all repair.
My darling says . . .'

My darling says nothing. Never, ever again.

Lilac in the jug on the table, the child asleep in the room across the hall, his even breathing coming in the silences between the songs, the night air through the open window from the yard outside. And then the words caught me unaware.

'The bridges break up in the panic of loss.'

That was it. The bridges broke. The walls collapsed. The dam ruptured and hopelessness flooded me. I stood in the brightly lit kitchen and wailed but no sound came. My body was churning, my throat choking but nothing came to cut out the sound of the words.

> 'Whither thou goest I will go
> And they turn as one and they head for the plain.'

And yet, on the face of it, morning was so different, so full of something else. Joy maybe, certainly forgetfulness, almost freedom. Almost because there is no such place. It doesn't exist. Once we've been through these sideroads there is no freedom from the memory of what we've seen or what we've done or what's been done to us. Certainly no freedom from things like this. From this thing.

In this morning's joy something snapped. Something said no. Something propelled me towards this song and undid all the years of distancing. How easily normality disintegrates. But how bright it was this morning. How hot the sun. How the lilacs swept in waves over the paths in the park. How certain the sycamores. And the red chestnut burning its candles. I swung the child in my arms, the child who is sleeping now, swung him like a little Icarus into the air and he spread his young wings and laughed and shouted, 'Again, again, do it again.' And I did, throwing him into the blue sheet of sky, catching him as he bounced back into my arms. 'Again,' he said. 'Do it again.'

And then I hoisted him into the dark places where the branches hide the secrets of childhood, into the shadows where the trees are. And he laughed in terror and delight. Higher than he had ever been and darker. Where he wanted to be. Where he feared. This child who is not mine was swinging wildly on the end of my arms, propelled where I had been propelled as a child, where I had propelled another child seven years ago. And his laugh was booming through the spaces between the trees. But it didn't strike me then. Maybe it should have done. There was just unease.

Whatever I've done in the past six months, with this child, I did before with that other, absent, child. Something made me uneasy but I couldn't pin it down. I just moved away and we went somewhere else.

'And he leans on her neck and he whispers low,
Whither thou goest I will go.'

But I can't, can I? I didn't. I didn't go where he went. And now I know what it was that sowed itself in my head this morning, what it was that waited all day for this song to release it.

That dark place in the branches, that sombre place where there is no sun, even in the height of summer. That cold place reminded me of the other cold black opening that I looked into and knew I was losing him. Wasn't that what terrified me, quietly? The unrelenting terror of shadow that will never lessen, the awful darkness that's real and imagined. Perhaps, in there, in the shades of the branches, he was waiting, watching this second betrayal. I didn't follow him into the first black pit and here I was with another child, playing as if nothing had ever happened, playing as if he had never existed. But he did. He does. Somewhere. Is it as close as that, as close as the shadows in the branches of summer trees? Or is it as far as the clammy silent place under six suffocating feet of clay? Or is it in the desperation of realization that some things are beyond cure, some situations are beyond rescue and his was one of them?

'At home on a branch in the highest tree,
A songbird sings out so suddenly.'

What did he carry with him into death, that small boy? Apart from terror? The knowledge that all the protection he saw in me was not enough. Fear. Maybe the knowledge that I wouldn't be there with him, even if I could be and who's to say I couldn't have gone? Who's to say we wouldn't have walked out together on some other side?

How easy it was to lie beside him on that bed, to hold on to him, to kiss his face and his hands. That was all so easy. And how easy to reassure him but he must have known, in one hope-less moment, that he was on his own, that boyhood, childhood, is no protection against being abandoned.

And what else did he take? One slight scar on his arm. The result of a joke that went suddenly wrong.

'Here,' I said, and I dipped the cooling iron against my palm. And then I glanced it against his skin. He was laughing, even as it burned his arm. I clattered it back on to the ironing board, the red welt rising on his skin.

'It's all right,' he said afterwards. 'It's all right, it was an accident.'

How often did I kiss that scar? Hundreds of times? Thousands? Not often enough.

'It's nearly better,' he said, a week afterwards, and he showed me the slight scar that will never go away.

> *'The bridges break up in the panic of loss*
> *And there's nothing to follow, there's no where to go.'*

Once the grave is closed there is no where to follow. There's no way through the shadows in the trees. But this is not a punish-ment, this is not your revenge, this isn't even that. It's my do-ing. And the tears won't come, only the dry retching that speaks of emptiness and promises emptiness. Forgive me, my son. Wait for me.

Wait for this man in the summer kitchen with the lilac closing as night comes on, this man haunted by the breathing of an-other child, this man who listens for some of the hope that was written into the song but cannot hear it.

> *'And the crickets are breaking his heart with their song,*
> *As the day caves in . . .'*

Extract from The Birds of the Innocent Wood

DEIRDRE MADDEN

At the moment when Jane's baby was born, she turned her head sharply aside to face the window, and as she felt the weight of the child slide from her body the physical pain receded. She opened her eyes and saw, through her tears, the flat lough burn up the golden light of an afternoon in early summer; the sky above the water was bleach-white. The scene was now so familiar to Jane that its very strangeness lay in its familiarity, like the sight of a loved one's half-remembered face, seen again after years of absence. She could scarcely have felt more amazed to open her eyes upon something completely unexpected; upon, say, a bright blue sea, or a forest filled with hunters and deer, than upon this stretch of predictable water.

'Don't you want to see your baby?' said the midwife's voice. 'It's a little boy.'

'No,' said Jane, and she quickly closed her eyes again upon the light of the view before her. The child had been stillborn: she had known that this would be so since the early stages of labour. Jane had resolved, even as she struggled to give birth, that she would not look at the baby.

'I don't want to see it, take it away please,' she said, her eyes still firmly closed.

But James wanted to see the child.

His presence at the confinement was precluded by the customs of that time and place, and on her arrival the midwife had bustled him out of the room. He was reluctant to leave. For some time after that he hovered around by the closed door, until the noises from within began to disturb him. The moans and half-whispers reminded him of the noises which he and Jane had once struggled to suppress so that his father would not hear them. He felt then that to listen at the door was wrong, and that he would either have to go into the room or go downstairs. For a moment he wanted to flout custom, to open the door and stay with Jane until the birth took place, if she would have him there. But his resolution wavered when he put his hand upon the doorknob: he could not bring himself to intrude upon the intimacy of what was already happening in the room, and sadly, reluctantly, he went down to the kitchen.

When the midwife told him what had happened, his first concern was for Jane. Assured of her health and safety, he then asked to see the child. The baby was brought to him and he looked at it: looked for a very long time. Then he swaddled the bundle up in his arms, and carried it upstairs. The midwife had told him of Jane's reluctance to look, but he wanted her to look too, and to be as amazed and comforted as he was. As soon as the bedroom door opened, however, and Jane caught sight of the white shawl, she hid her head under the blankets.

'Take it away from me,' she said. 'It's dead, and I won't look at it.'

'He's a lovely baby,' said James, 'and you ought at least to look at him. You'll regret it later if you don't.'

The muffled voice from under the blankets said again, 'Take it away from me. Take it away.'

James did not reply, but he left the room. When the door closed and she could hear the sound of his feet descending the stairs, Jane poked her head out above the blankets. She lay there alone for a long time, and by dusk she had drifted off into a deep and dreamless sleep.

She awoke in darkness. Night had long since fallen, and while she slept, someone had pulled the curtains and had tucked the blankets neatly up around her, but in her first moments of consciousness, this was not what Jane noticed. Instead, she felt instinctively that something was wrong, something was different, something more than the absence of James from her side. And then she realized: for months now she had been woken daily not by the light of morning, nor by a clock, nor by James calling her because it was time to rise and work: she had been roused by the baby who woke independently and, floating inside her, kicked her into consciousness. Now her body was still and quiet as an empty house; the baby was gone. Very quietly she began to cry. The bedroom door was slightly ajar, and between the noise of her sobs she could hear the steady and unbroken beat of the big clock in the hall. Time was a trap, coiled like a spring around her, and she could see a life open out beyond her, hours, days, weeks, months, years, spiralling away to her own death, and she would have to live that life.

Every point of apparent change would be just a point of variation, moving her into the next circle of her existence, which would be not quite the same as the preceding circle, but which would be a circle still. It was a long time before she slept again.

Two days later, the baby was buried: not in the family grave with his grandparents, but alone at the foot of the hill. When Jane was told this, she closed her eyes and she did not speak. She felt the last possible shred of comfort melt away from her, and she knew as a cold fact that she would never be whole again, that this final cruelty had broken something in her which could never be mended.

She came downstairs for the first time seven days later. Her body as she dressed felt curiously flat and light, but she moved much more slowly and deliberately than she had ever done during her pregnancy. When she appeared at the kitchen door James, who was sitting drinking tea at the table, looked up in surprise. He had been encouraging her to rise for some days now, but she had given no indication that she would do so. He smiled at her, but she did not return the smile. She crossed in silence to the armchair beside the stove, and sat down.

'Would you like a cup of tea? There's some left in the pot.'

She shook her head.

'Is there anything I can get for you?'

Again the same response, and then Jane fixed her gaze on a point in the middle distance, somewhere past James's head. While she looked away, James continued to drink his tea and watch her, until suddenly he realized that this was how it had all started in that café, four years ago. He wondered now what he would have said if, on that day, someone had told him of all that was to happen between them, and that yet, four years later, they would be sitting together in an identical pose, as if nothing whatever had changed, as if they were still strangers and in each other's company by mere chance of circumstance.

He remembered that day vividly and with guilt, for what had interested him first in Jane was a self-possession so complete that it withdrew all feeling and all personality from her face, and he felt that he was looking at a mask: a familiar mask. The large blue eyes, the high forehead, the pale skin: these features formed a face which was, to James, so passive and lifeless, that as he watched, he found himself grafting on a personality and a past life which belonged to someone else, but which, oddly, seemed to fit.

He was so absorbed in this task that when the young woman at last turned to him and spoke, he was shocked and quickly became confused. He knew that he had done something wrong. He engaged her in conversation and listened politely when she spoke, as though to give some credit to the reality of her personality. He remembered the horrible little tingle of fear he had felt when the woman lowered her eyes and with seeming artlessness told him the story of her life; for it was no more than a variation of the life he had given her. When she stood up to leave he felt a sense of panic: if he lost her now, for the rest of his life he would wonder if she was real, knew that soon he might believe her to be nothing more than a creature of his imagination, conjured up out of his unhappiness and loneliness. So he had quickly asked to see her again: Jane had said, 'Yes.'

Often since that day he wished that when she finished her tea and rose to leave the café, he had said no more than 'Goodbye.' Often since that day little instances of her lack of feeling had horrified him. He had tried to understand the misery of her loneliness, and the strange, sad life which had made her the woman she was. But as he looked at her now, sitting stiffly in the chair beside the stove, he knew that her new grief would do nothing to soften her. She had put herself beyond the power of his comfort, and she would keep herself rigidly there; nor could she be a comfort to him. And James felt a great sense of pity which encompassed them both as he looked at her, and remembered that they would be husband and wife until death.

In the following weeks, their lives began to get back into some semblance of order. Jane found that the routine chores of the farm allowed her to slip back into a life identical to the life which she had lived since first coming to the house. She went through many of the motions and emotions which she had experienced at the time of her father-in-law's death, and her sadness now was that the baby had left so little mark upon the house: there was so little to be done. Over a year ago she had cleared out the old man's cluttered bedroom, and had been amazed to think that all these things would never be needed again. Now, she had to dismantle the nursery which she had so carefully prepared.

She remembered sorting through her father-in-law's clothes, remembered the strange intimacy of that, for they smelt of sweat and tobacco, they were creased and the cuffs were grimy, and they would never be any more smelly, crumpled or dirty than they were then. But now she was faced with another pile of clothes to be disposed of, and although their owner was dead too, the pain here was that the clothes were all perfect, all clean, untouched, unworn. There were thick piles of soft white nappies, little jackets and hats and boots, most of which she had herself knitted, and a long white christening robe, the newness of which she resented most of all. The clothes were all so soft and tiny that it seemed ludicrous, unbelievable, that their owner could be dead. Dead people were old people, people like parents who had worn out their clothes, their bodies, their lives. Kneeling by the side of the bed, she buried her face in the heap of baby clothes, feeling their softness and wishing that they could be pervaded with the warm, milky, sexless smell of a baby, but she knew that they would never be; knew that there would never be anything more than this smell of newness and clean wool. People in the village said to her that she was young, she would have another child, but that did nothing to placate her. She could not yet bear to think of the possibility of having another baby, of going through all that long waiting again, perhaps to face at last that same sadness and disappointment. But even if she did have another baby, she knew that she would never again have *that* baby, the baby who was dead. And these clothes belonged to that baby: she felt that it would be a violation to allow another child to wear them.

One afternoon in July, she lit a fire in the yard, and then, one by one, she carefully fed each little garment into the flames. When they were all gone, she realized that the only material proof she now had that the baby had ever existed were two pieces of paper: one a birth certificate, one a death certificate. There were also some little silvery stretch marks upon her body.

James was angry about the burning of the clothes. She had thought that he might be, and so she made a point of doing it while he was out across the fields working, and also of telling him what she had done as soon as he came back to the farm. He was angry, hurt and angry; and these were the responses she had expected and desired. They were back again at the point to which they had been brought by the death of his father: they had no one but each other. Now, however, Jane did not want to cling to him, but to wound him. Since that first death she felt that they had become truly married; felt that he was a part of her and she was a part of him, and so she now wanted to hurt and wound him because she wanted to hurt and wound herself. Seeing his pain, and seeing that she worsened it, gave her a bleak form of satisfaction.

One day in July when she went out to the byre to call him for lunch, she found him weeping. She did nothing to comfort him. Although she wanted to go over to him and embrace him, wanted to do that more than anything else in the world, she beat this feeling down, and she stood there in silence, coldly watching him. She saw that he was ashamed of his tears, and that her silence only made his weeping sound the more pathetic and weak. At last, still crying, he pushed past her out of the byre and across the yard.

Jane, of course, also cried: often she would be engaged on some simple chore in the house and think that her sadness was not worse than any other time, when suddenly whatever was before her—a basin of potatoes which she happened to be peeling, or a piece of mending on which she was engaged—these things would suddenly blur and vanish before her unexpected tears. When this happened she did not seek out her husband, but fell back on the perverse strength of her childhood, and hid herself away until she had willed herself over this brief loss of face.

One morning when they were sitting in silence at breakfast, James suddenly said to Jane, 'It's not my fault that the baby died, you know. I'm not to blame.'

Jane did not reply. The tense atmosphere was not eased by the arrival of Gerald some moments later. Without him ever saying so, it was evident throughout that summer that his own marriage with Ellen was proving to be intensely unhappy. Jane noticed this, but it barely surprised her, and she did not care. Her own misery kept her fully occupied, and the same was true of James, who did not have the necessary strength both to bear his loss and to humour Jane. Perhaps he did not realize that she needed to be humoured, for he did not understand the nature of her grief, did not understand that she was translating it into anger and deflecting it on to him. Her anger, her coldness, her sullenness made James feel hurt and resentful. By the time summer was at its height, relations between them were worse than they had ever been before.

Jane's resentment of her husband grew in proportion to her regret that she had not looked at the child; and that regret grew fast, until it soon reached the point of obsession. Night after night she would dream about the baby. In her dreams the child was sitting upon her lap and facing away from her, but when she tried to make him turn his head, the child strongly resisted. At last she would succeed, only to find nothing: only to find that the front of the child's head was as blank as that of a tailoress's dummy. She began to cry, and then the faceless baby vanished.

She envied James because he had looked at the baby, and hated herself because she had not. She was too proud to ask him to describe the child to her, and also too wretched. She knew that no matter what he said, it would never be enough; that the mystery would always remain, and there was no one she could blame for this but herself. Even with this knowledge, she spent hours leafing through a book about childcare, looking intently at each of the photographs. Once, she even went to the city on the pretext of making a shopping trip, but she spent the day walking around, looking at all the babies and trying to imagine the variations necessary in each face to create the face of her own lost child. It was, of course, a futile exercise, and left her frustrated and unhappy.

She was deeply hurt, too, by the child's exclusion from the family grave, and his relegation to the patch of ground at the foot of the hill. In the course of that summer, she spent many hours thinking about this. She realized that she would never be buried with her child unless she took her own life.

One night she could not sleep, and lay awake for hours beside James. She thought about the baby: once, it had had a place in time. As she listened to James's steady breathing, she remembered the time after his father's death when they had been happy together, remembered the nights of the preceding summer, during one of which the baby had been conceived, and tried to understand how the child had passed so quickly from that physical reality to its present state. She wanted to understand this as far as she possibly could, and rising from the warmth of the bed, she left the room. Barefoot and wearing only her thin nightdress, Jane went downstairs and passed through the empty house, opened the back door and walked out into the night. She stopped in the middle of the yard, and turned her face away from the lough shore, on the far side of which she could see a few yellow lights twinkle; turned too from the house. Instead, she put back her head and looked up at the sky, which was moonless and starless and black. She tried to imagine the baby in just such a blackness, but this was not a void, and she could not properly imagine a soul beyond help, beyond time, beyond reach, for she could feel a light breeze upon her face and the ground under her feet was hard and cold; the leaves rustled in the orchard and she could hear the cries of the birds; when she breathed in she could smell the earth's dampness. Then she knew that she would never be able to take her own life, that it was a thing too terrible and too sacred. Death did not end life, it merely changed it. She knew that she would never be able to believe anything other than this. The baby was still real, but it was in a reality outside time.

For the rest of that summer, Jane waited. She knew what was going to happen, but did not know the precise moment when the consciousness of everything around her would overwhelm her completely. James, in retrospect, would think that during that summer she had withdrawn into herself, that she had cut herself off from the world, when in fact the exact opposite was true. Never before had she felt so vulnerable and open to the mere existence of other things. When she looked at an animal or a flower, her own identity dissolved and flowed out, so that she could hardly tell where she, Jane, ended, and the cat or the rose began. Her mind felt raw as a wound, every thought a touch that hurt. The presence of Gerald and James did not really register with her, but she watched obsessively all the natural things around her. She waited for summer to end and the autumn to come, longing for this to happen, even though the knowledge of what it would bring frightened her.

All the flowers in the garden died, and the air at night became cool and sharp. She watched the swallows as they crowded along the telegraph wires, strung out like plain-chant against the white sky. Jane watched them do this for several days, and then one morning she awoke to find the wires all bare, for the birds had flown away. She felt completely abandoned.

Later that day, she accidentally broke a white dinner plate. It cracked cleanly in two, and she held up the two halves in her hands, looking at them as though they were the first things she had understood in months.

When James returned from the cottage that evening, he found

that the farm was apparently deserted. He looked for Jane in every room, then searched around the farm-yard, but he did not find her. He went back into the house and was standing in the kitchen wondering what to do next, when he heard a noise in the hallway. He listened again, and it led him to the cupboard under the stairs, where he found her curled up with her hands across her face. She would not look at him, and she would not speak. When he tried to make her leave the cupboard, she resisted him strongly.

Until the year had almost ended, they kept her in an asylum which reeked of disinfectant and polish. James visited her frequently, and for the first month Jane treated him as she had on the day when he found her under the stairs, refusing either to look at him or to speak. The doctors told him that she wanted to stay in darkness and silence at all times, and cried like a child when she was forced into the light or was questioned.

After a few weeks, her condition appeared to improve. She became more tractable, and when James visited she would talk with him, although with excessive politeness and formality. The treatment she received made her forgetful, and James found it upsetting, frightening even, when she failed to remember things which he had told her on earlier visits.

'You must be making a mistake,' she would say quietly. 'You never told me that before now.' And to humour her he would tell it all again, only to find on successive visits that she had still no recollection of his conversations. Once she became angry, and said that he was deliberately telling her lies to try to confuse her, and thereafter he gave in to her completely: yes, it was he who was forgetful; no, he had never told her such and such a thing until now. But it did frighten him to talk to her and see her watch him as though with piercing clarity, while knowing that she was absorbing nothing of what was being said to her. He was told that she had become very religious, so he was surprised when she said, 'Before I come home, I want you to take down all the holy pictures in the house, and put them away somewhere that I won't find them.' James promised that he would do this, and the following week she again made the same request and again he made his promise, although he had already put all the pictures and statues up in the attic. Jane frowned and pressed her palms together. 'They might let me home in time for Christmas, if I'm a good girl,' she said, with such extreme artlessness that James, knowing Jane, could not help but believe the remark was veined with irony, her illness notwithstanding.

'That would be good, wouldn't it?' he said.

'Yes.' She paused for a moment, then said again, 'You will put the pictures away before I get home, won't you?'

'Yes, of course.'

'I had a dream and it was very hot, I was suffocating and the pain, you wouldn't believe the pain, I was all sweating and blood and the pain, there were little flies all around my face and I couldn't brush them away, my eyes kept closing and I knew that if I didn't keep them open I would close them once and never open them again.' Again she was silent, and twisted her palms together. 'Before Christmas. Perhaps. If I'm good.'

Exactly a week before Christmas, James collected Jane and took her home. As they drove towards the farm, they saw Ellen in the distance, and making no comment, Jane instinctively turned her head aside, and did not look up again until they had driven past the woman. She did not see, therefore, that Ellen was pregnant. James had not dared to tell her this while she was ill, and the sight of Ellen on the road had terrified him until he saw Jane pointedly look away. Still, he dreaded the day when she would find out. She was bound to know eventually.

As they drew up at the door of the farm, Jane was thinking of the day when first she came to the house, when she had been startled by the clamour of the wild birds, for she had expected only silence. The wildness of the landscape had frightened her, but in the years which had passed since that day she had been frightened even more by that which she had found in herself. She felt ashamed to think that she had been that stupid girl, who had come to the house with all her hopes and her expectations. She did not believe that a single illusion was left, and she was grateful for that.

'Are you glad to be home?'

'Yes.'

Jane walked through all the rooms of the house, touching things and smelling them, looking pointedly at the rectangles of unfaded wallpaper where the holy pictures had been hanging, but she made no comment.

She went to bed early that night, for she was very tired. James soon followed her, and found that she was already lying tucked up. He undressed and got into bed beside her, leaning over to kiss her in a rather hesitant way upon the cheek. Her skin smelt of soap.

'I'm so glad that you're home and that you're well again,' he said.

She smiled and settled down stiffly, lying far from him at the edge of the bed. After he put out the light, however, she said, 'Give me your hand please.' And when he did she gripped it tightly. They fell asleep thus, hand in hand and side by side, lying flat in the dark, as a dead knight and his lady carved in stone might lie upon their tomb for centuries, in the still and silent darkness of an empty chapel.

Extract from Who Trespass Against Us

In September 1990 our eldest son, Peter, was killed in a car accident. In three weeks he would have been sixteen. During 1991–2 I wrote Who Trespass Against Us *from which this extract is taken.*

While our grief has become part of the permanent texture of our lives, Peter's death is a continuing powerful catalyst for our personal enrichment.

Time was neither friend nor enemy to Adam, neither rigid nor plastic. Zoe had died a lifetime ago in the last few seconds the year after the year after next. People came and went below him like faces passing a reviewing stand. An undertaker who said, 'Sorry to have met you, sorry.' At the grave, ten or a dozen young men and women, Zoe's friends, some of whom shook his hand, and his father, Pom, out of place, embarrassed evidence of natural order stood on its head, floating along like someone hired for the day from a waxworks.

Standing in his house, in a room swirling with people, Adam saw Danny O'Malley angling for him.

'Adam.'

Danny was a very big man, as big as Adam. He manoeuvred Adam into a bear hug. 'Adam, I don't want you to say anything, but what I have to say can be said in a minute. Zoe is alright, okay? I know this. We are the ones in pain. I knew today in that church, at that grave, that Zoe is happy. She's laughing! She's praying for us, Adam. She's lucky because she's free. Beyond hurt, alright? We're hurting. I say we, of course I mean you, because my hurt is a bruise but yours is a massive gash, an amputation, an arm—you know?—a leg, gone, it can't grow back, but the hurt won't always be there. Zoe is always there. She's with Christ. She's so . . . so lucky! We're unlucky. We're left in a deep hole that we can't get out of. But if you look up you can see the sky! Christ is the sky, Adam. Find Christ and you will find what you have lost and the courage you need to go on. I love you.'

'Danny . . .'

He hid from them in Zoe's room. With its long-forgotten music contemporanea it was really the room of Zoe years ago, of Zoe before she left. The bed seemed small as he lay on it, his feet propped on the endboard, staring as she must have done at the sky, looking for some sign. Everything was gut. Blood boiled and pounded, the sky he knew was blue he saw through a prism rinded. Exhausted by his sheer inability to attempt understanding, he began to search for clues to what had happened in Alison, his wife.

She was different. She had left him in the pew that morning and when she asked from the lectern in a voice rock steady, 'Death, where is thy sting?', the great yearning for such strength among the gathering of casual believers had been palpable. She had caught his hand when he came in from Barts and said: 'Poor Adam.' Other women in the room had wept but Alison's face had shone with the brittleness of shells. He and she had entered a new world whose creation had come with the first news of Zoe's death. Everything had changed, had become unendurable.

The Garden of Eden

EILÍS NÍ DHUIBHNE

*This story was written during a mood of loss and loneliness
in a garden on an August day. I think my children were away
from home at the time. I have, luckily, never lost a child but,
like many mothers, often dread that possibility.*

In the end, David simply said, 'I am going.' And Carmelita
knew what he meant.

'All right,' she replied. She had been waiting for this announce-
ment for twelve years. She had feared it, postponed it, protested
against it, and also, at other times, of course wanted it, craved it,
paved the way for it. Now, this now, this minute, sitting, appro-
priately, at the kitchen table (*ad mensa*. What's the Latin for
'at', she wondered idly), it was nothing but a bald fact, like the
sun that shone on the lawn outside, like the marigold in the
window-box, like the wine-glass of water on the blue checked
cloth.

David stood up, leaving a little food on his plate, and went
upstairs. Carmelita sat, gazing absently out the window. The
laburnum was dropping black pods on the yard. The lobelia
had withered. A few montbretiae bloomed with their character-
istic brilliance in the euphemistically named rockery but mostly
the garden was on the wane. Middle August, and hardly a thing
left in it. After nine years in the house. And garden. David usu-
ally took care of the garden. The split would be mainly *ad hortis*,
actually, she thought calmly, pleased to remember this word, if
not its cases. He'd never done anything much at the table ex-
cept eat the food she'd cooked.

Carmelita considered the garden next door as she often did. It
was the horticultural *tour de force* of the neighbourhood: tender
velvet lawn, bright but not gaudy borders, shrubs in all the
right corners, flowering or leafing in a happy sequence of col-
ours, scents and textures. Patio, arbour, roses clambering over
trellis, geraniums in great carved terracotta pots. An ornate Vic-

torian conservatory.

Carmelita envied them, those next door. She coveted that garden. She craved it passionately.

David popped his head in and said: 'I'm off now. Goodbye!' His heavy step sounded on the hall floor. The door opened and then shut slowly and sadly, but firmly.

Carmelita stopped thinking about the garden next door. She got up and plugged in the kettle and made a cup of tea. When it was ready, she carried it out to the garden, her own garden, and sat down at the table there. A white plastic table with a green sun umbrella, and a few odd, mismatched lawnchairs surrounding it. She sat and looked at her shrubs, her flowers, her trees, and the sky. The evening sky in early autumn, the middle ages of the year. The little bit she could see in the gap between the sycamores was a pale wishy washy pink. The sun had already disappeared behind the roofs of the houses on the next road. The summer is over, well and truly over, she thought and a dreadful last-rose-of summer sentiment of loss and bereavement overwhelmed her for a few minutes. But she did not wallow in it; she waited for it to pass, because she was so accustomed to this sensation.

Periodically, every year from about the tenth of August to the beginning of September it struck. Her last-rose-of-summer depression. She was very sensitive to seasonal cycles, like a lot of women who live in suburbs. The beginning of nice ones, like spring or summer, brought jubilance. The end of nice ones— and there is only one season that really ends—was like a great tragedy which experience seemed to exaggerate rather than assuage. And August seemed much more of an ending, so much gloomier, than September, which had its own character and self-confidence and was the beginning of something again, even if it was something not very good. School. Frost. Long dark nights.

Carmelita and David had been married for twelve years. Oh yes! How time flew. It seemed no length at all since their wedding. Since that time of being in love with David. Perhaps time does not exist when the emotions are concerned. On the other hand it was aeons ago; its trappings belonged to history. That ceremony in the registry office in Kildare Street. The drinks afterwards in the Shelbourne, with everyone dressed up somehow. The bridesmaid in white pants and a navy striped t-shirt had looked odd, certainly. Carmelita could have killed her. But most of them had made a respectable effort with flowery dresses and hats. Outmoded. Dated. Ancient.

David had been as always: smiling broadly, jocular and in full control. He was smart and quick witted, David. She had basked in that, in this protection. He was never at a loss. His decisions were, almost invariably, the correct ones. And he never regretted them, as a matter of principle.

The decision to get married had not been his, of course, but hers. And her decisions were frequently wrong, she had found out as her life progressed. Usually they were irrational, whereas David's would as a rule be the opposite. It had seemed terribly necessary to marry him at that time twelve years ago, though. She had been pregnant, but that was not why. It had seemed necessary before the pregnancy, which was an effect, not a cause, of the need. Marriage to David had seemed to be her only salvation, the only course open to her in life. Life without him, she thought, was unthinkable. She would die without him. She would wither up and cease to exist.

And indeed her expectations had been fulfilled. Marriage had brought happiness and activity. Life had been full as a tick. It ticked, ticked all day, all night. There was never a moment's idleness. She had been so busy, so very busy, for several years. So busy that she had not time to consider whether she was happy or not.

Only in retrospect did she realise how happy she had been during that hectic time. Not having time to think of it, that had been her happiness, it seemed. Not having time to bless herself.

She was not busy any more.

The garden was empty before her eyes. Friday evening. She had the weekend free, three nights, two whole days, all for herself.

She walked over to the fence dividing her garden from the

garden of Eden. She did this every night, because the neighbours were away on their fortnight's holiday in Greece. There was a broken place on the fence—God knows how they had let it remain broken—over which she could peer and get a perfect view.

The first sight of it broke upon her like a peaceful oriental vision: there was a quietness in this garden, partly because it was quiet since there was nobody in it, but more because of its perfection. The greenest grass. The fluid forms of the bushes. The pale pinks, yellows, lilacs of the flowers. It was in no way a busy garden, although it required much business to achieve the effect it created. Like a beautiful, rich room, upon which endless attention and expense has been lavished, it looked natural and spontaneous.

David had driven off in the car. She had heard him starting it, she remembered, just after the door shut. He was possibly far away by now. The thought that there was no longer a car crossed her mind, like a slight shadow, and disappeared. Who needs a car?

She began to climb the fence. A thin wooden fence. It was not difficult, because it had wires attached to it, bits of broken chicken wire up which she had once tried to grow woodbine but without success.

She swung herself over the narrow top and jumped on to the pale red pavingstones of the patio next door. At first she stood and looked around at everything she had seen so often from the other side of the fence. The palm and elephant grass just where the patio met the lawn. The green hose lying on the slabs. The pots of deeply pink geraniums all around. And, placed at interesting vantage points further down the garden, beds of lupins, hollyhocks, columbines and canterbury bells, their colours deep and velvet, their heads bowing, one to the other, like coquettish ladies at some brilliantly flirtatious court. She breathed deeply, and perfume from mignonette, honeysuckle and escallonia filled her lungs, along with a headier, more intoxicating air: something like incense.

She walked slowly along the lawn. The greenness of it soaked into her skin; she could feel her body absorbing it. It was like swimming softly, breaststroking through a long aquamarine pool. Or through a cloud. Although naturally she had never swum in a cloud.

She sat on the grass for a minute. It was dampish. She could feel the wet seeping into her skirt. A ladybird came and crawled along her leg, one of the more unusual yellow ladybirds which, in their gay spotted shells, reminded Carmelita of fashionably rigged-out toddlers. It was a great year for these insects. All the gardens were infested with them. They were tolerated even by the best gardeners on account of their appetite for greenflies. All years were great years for greenfly.

Carmelita stayed on the grass for a long time. Then she got up and left using the same route and technique she'd employed in entry. Before she left she cut three slips from the geraniums, whose pink blossoms rested like hot fluttering butterflies on their turgid foliage. And when she got to her own side of the fence, she potted the slips in terracotta plastic pots, in peat moss, and put them on the window sill to root. She had heard from a woman she'd met once on a plane to London that stolen slips did best.

She went to bed. The house creaked a lot. Some doors banged because a window was open. She thought about burglars. She believed in burglars, but her image of them, like her childhood images of God and the Devil, was vague. They were male, they would break glass, they would burst into her bedroom and . . .

Lulled by such creaks and bangs and ideas, she fell asleep.

The next day would have been long and empty, had she not decided in the morning that she really must go shopping. So she took the bus into the city centre and spent the whole day walking around the shops, trying on clothes, examining furniture and rugs. Time passes very quickly in town, and she remembered the Saturdays of her youth, her later youth that is, when she had lived with her mother and had her job, the job she still had. Shop after shop, garment after garment. Bought, worn a few times, discarded.

She bought a white linen suit. And a bag of peaches. And a packet of incense sticks.

And several small terracotta pots.

That evening, she watched television and cut three slips of escallonia in the garden next door.

She burned incense, thinking how David hated incense or anything that seemed cheap and eastern, like curried eggs and the novels of Hesse and Indian rugs. She drank some red wine but it was sour as it usually is if you buy a cheap bottle in a supermarket and she could not take more than one glass.

Her thoughts were less of burglars as she lay in bed, and more of the past. Not the past with David, which hardly seemed like past. But of her childhood, of her teenage years which seemed, in retrospect, serene and carefree. She also thought about her slips and planned the future of her garden. Every mickle makes a muckle, she thought, and eventually it will look like theirs next door. Patience is a virtue.

Carmelita was not an especially patient woman, and on Sunday she went to a garden centre and bought a palm tree and a blue hydrangea (she'd never fancied the pink) and came home and planted them on the back lawn. And that night, after dark, she stole a large carved terracotta pot from the garden next door. But for the time being she put it in her bedroom where the next-door neighbours were not likely to see it.

That night as she lay in bed she thought of the next-door neighbours. They would not have seen the pot if she'd put it in the hall or the living-room either, she thought, because they did not visit her house. The reason was, she and David had had such fearful rows in the year or two after the accident. Carmelita had been given to screaming loudly in the middle of the night. She used to accuse David of all kinds of awful things: not being sensitive, not caring about her, not giving the love she needed. She had ranted and raved and screamed at the top of her voice, and sometimes David had hit her. To shut her up. Battered. She had been a battered wife, according to a certain point of view. In her own estimation, in retrospect but even at the time, she could justify David's hitting her. They always say they've been provoked. But in his case it was, she suspected, true. Anyway invariably she had hit him back, and not infrequently she had hit him first. They had been like two boys scuffling in the school playground.

Except that the sound effects were higher pitched and more alarming.

They heard. She knew they must have heard. It was so embarrassing. She hadn't wanted to speak to them. She didn't speak to them, or have cups of tea with them, or invite them in for a drink on Christmas Eve.

It had all stopped long ago. There was no noise, no screaming. No fighting at all. But the pattern was set. No neighbourliness. No visits.

Lulled by these thoughts she fell asleep.

The next morning was Monday and Carmelita was supposed to get up and go to work. She worked in a bank. She was a cashier. It was not as boring to her now as it had been when she'd started it: she enjoyed saying hello to the customers, she liked to be nice and friendly and make them feel at ease, which is not how most people feel in a bank. And also, over the years, she had grown fond of her colleagues and of her salary.

But this morning she did not go to work. She got up at the usual time of eight o'clock and went down and had her coffee. But when the time for leaving the house came, she did not go. Instead she went into the garden. She examined the slips: none of them had withered so far, which she took to be a good sign. Now she had fuchsia, escallonia, and geraniums on the go. She climbed over the fence and looked around. The garden next door looked even more wonderful than usual in the early morning light. The fresh clean sunshine, the unsullied air of start of day, suited its own spick and span, cared for character. It was in its element.

Carmelita walked all around it, simply admiring. She no longer felt any envy or covetousness, she realised, and supposed it must be because she knew that soon—or at least eventually—she was going to have her own beautiful garden. As beautiful as this. Or more beautiful? No. Just the same.

What would she take? She remembered that they were due home the day after tomorrow, so her time in the garden was limited, and she would have to choose exactly what she wanted now. She looked at dahlias, and lupins, and tearoses. Broom and rose of sharon and a shrub she did not know the name of which had greenish reddish leaves and huge fluffy red balls. She looked at elephant grass and marram grass and cordyline.

In the end, she cried, 'Ah!' Because she saw it. Just exactly what she had wanted all the time. How odd that she had not seen it before; how very odd. In the corner of the patio, propped up against the wall, was a small tricycle belonging to the youngest child next door. There were three children, two girls and a boy. The boy was the youngest. He was four, and this was his bicycle.

She grabbed it and let it down over the fence as gently as she could. Then she herself climbed over, and carried the tricycle up to her bedroom, where she put it on the floor just beside the bed.

After the accident, all Raymond's things had been given away. Absolutely everything: David had thought it was better that way. It was all as bad as it could be. They didn't need reminders, he had said, packing the toys and the clothes and things, Raymond's things, into boxes for the travellers who called to the door every Saturday, regular as clockwork.

There were the photographs, of course, but only in albums. None out on the sideboard, none displayed with the other photographs on the mantelpiece. They had to get over it. They had to forget.

She lay in bed for a while, thinking about her slips and glancing at the tricycle from time to time. Then she searched in the drawers of David's desk for the albums. She selected three of the nicest pictures, showing Raymond at one, three and seven and a half, just after he'd made his First Communion and just before he'd died. She propped them up on her dressing table where she could see them at night before going to sleep and in the morning as soon as she awoke. She'd get some frames for them later. Later today, or maybe tomorrow, or maybe she'd ask David to get them.

Because of course he was going to come back.

And David came back that very night, because he'd rung the office and she hadn't been there, and because he couldn't cook, and for various other reasons. His decisions were usually rational, and usually correct, and he hardly ever regretted them, on principle.

Extract from Memories of Snow

ALISON DYE

This piece is a letter from an American woman to her dead son, three years after he has been killed in World War II. Not long before I was born, my mother's oldest brother died in much the same circumstances as the young man in the book. My grandparents' loss of their first child, my mother's loss of her beloved brother, brought a terrible grieving into our family which has wept like an open wound into the generations, the enormity of Eric's absence and the circumstances that brought it about almost too much to bear or take in. Like the young man in the book, Eric could not be brought home for burial, and remains in the American Military Cemetery in Henri Capelle, Belgium.

20 December, 1949. 3.00 a.m.

Dear Johnny,

It seems strange, writing to you again after so long. I'm sorry, but I had to give it up. It was when we got word that you were gone and like with Joe we had no money to bring you home. As I am writing this now I seem to be speaking of a time that happened to someone else. And yet if I feel nothing, why do I want to beg your forgiveness for leaving you in Belgium? President Roosevelt died that same year, in April, and I could hardly go on, the grief over this man consumed us all, oh, we understood what had happened to him.

I stopped writing because I couldn't take any more thinking about you. Please don't misunderstand, I don't really mean that the way it sounds, of course I wanted to think about you and I wanted with all my heart to have you back. It's just that I would go days and days accomplishing nothing, failing everyone around me, going over and over what went wrong, the bad decisions I made, how young you were. My mind had become a racing engine that wouldn't stop, there were days I was out of control of my own mind, Johnny. I was unable to meet my responsibilities, and that is not right, that is not my way—I hope you understand. Once in a while I would get a break, I would find myself wondering about the bake sale at church, or the blouse I was sewing for Lizzie, and then suddenly I would say to myself, Hazel, there you go now, you weren't thinking about Johnny! Why, the worst must be over, you'll get on with living now! I can tell you I had to give myself a good talking to many times. But to think this is what I had come to, trying to will my own child out of my life, the nights and mornings I wept. The knowledge that you would never come back to us was like a vice tightening and crushing me. I was ashamed of shedding those tears when I knew that in the end I would have to turn my back on you and get on with what little life we had left. God forgive me.

So I would go along and begin to think I was past you, and then a bit of news would come along and I'd want to tell you— Bert and Sadie's new calf—and I'd sit down again to write, saying oh, I know he's gone, for goodness sake, it's just a letter, it doesn't mean anything, and before long I'd be fighting the truth again, getting nowhere, my mind so mad at the Army, the Germans, the bad weather in Belgium, my own careless, unforgiveable judgement to have let you go when my duty was to protect you. Even now, right this minute I ask myself: Hazel, *what were you thinking?* A child in a war? What was the matter with you? And when my mind goes this way I am right back where I started, I read and re-read your last letters, the early letters, trying to turn back the clock—I even smashed the clock Granddad gave you. What a thing to do, to blame a clock! I'm sorry, Johnny, I know it meant a lot to you. But there it is, I did it, the incessant ticking was a torture, a knife stabbing me, my rational mind could not overcome it. But of course afterwards I was nowhere nearer to accepting things, nowhere nearer my own life. What is my own life? The girls who came back from their war jobs, they would laugh at me, they seem to laugh at everyone now. They wore men's overalls in the factories, did men's jobs, went against everything their Christian upbringing taught them, pretending all the while they cared only for you boys, but we saw the pictures of them in *Life* Magazine, smiling, their hair in a bob.

Well, now they're back and they want 'rights', freedom, I don't know what they're talking about. The world is all changed, Johnny, you wouldn't recognise it yourself, and I don't even know what I mean by all the things I try to say to myself. Like: go on living, Hazel. The past is over, you had a certain life before, now that's done and you'll have a different life, you could be happy in a different way. But in my letters, in my mind, I tell you about the *old* life—it's the only one that seems to make sense to me. But certain events have happened and so I have to stop that life, I must do it once and for all and that is why I am writing to you today. So early in the morning and I cannot sleep. I see that it will snow soon, it has been a bitter winter. I must keep to my determination to write this letter. I am sorry to have to tell you what I have become. . . .

And now I will tell you what I did last night, after I knew Raymond was gone, after I had been unable to see him. Then I will leave you in peace—for I know this is a burden to you, because like me, you had no experience of the world. We thought we did and we thought it was all we needed to know. Please hear me out, I am not proud of myself, but I want it said. After Dad and Billy were asleep and I was alone in the living room, I threw all my old letters to you into the fire. I tore them up like an insane person, my hands were shaking with the grief and fury I was in, I had become someone else—it wasn't me and yet I was the only one there, driven by a force beyond my power to stop, tearing those letters and sobbing, throwing feeble bits of paper at a roaring fire, and even then having the memory—shocking myself at what a sweetness suddenly came to me for I have been incapable of the slightest tenderness—the memory of you and Raymond trying to teach me to throw a baseball! I could never get it right! You were so patient with me, so grown-up. And last night as I stood face to face with that fire, I threw with all my might just the way you always said I should—let go and throw with everything you've got, Ma! you used to say—and I felt I was throwing every dream Dad and I ever had into that blaze and I was crying There! There! Take him! Take all of them! Go ahead! I was not in control of my thoughts, Johnny, something carried me away from all reason and common sense, and then I tore open the letters from you, those bright letters from the Front, when everything was fine. You were full of hope and courage and pride! One at a time I ripped them apart in a frenzy, and I screamed Lies! Lies! and pushed them at the fire, stuffed them deep into the fire, kicked the logs, the sparks flew up like explosions, and at that moment I did not feel the burns on my hands and feet, but now I feel the pain and I am glad of it, the crimson skin is stiff and raw and throbbing, this torment is the only thing in me that remains alive, the agony of these burns, and if this goes away, I will do it again, and again and again, such a searing wretchedness is what I have become. The shame of it, to have to reveal the darkness I never knew lurked and crept in my soul. But I see now there is no avoiding the mention of things as they are. Where did I go wrong? Can anyone tell me?

This is the place where time and events have brought us.

This is the trail we have left behind.

I am a cold person now, Johnny. I don't mean to be, it's not what I planned, you must be somewhere in my heart, surely a mother cannot forget her own child, surely a living human being cannot turn to stone and ice.

Perhaps someday I will be able to find us both again.

Good-bye.

Extract from An Ordinary Hero

ALF McCREARY

This biography of Gordon Wilson was written with the full support of Mrs Joan Wilson and the family, following many long interviews. I believe that this process was helpful in dealing with their bereavement, in the same way that my work on an earlier publication on the death of Marie Wilson had given Gordon himself an opportunity to talk about and to share his deep personal loss.

Gordon, Joan and Peter, who was now a toddler, moved from the flat over the drapery shop to what is still the Wilson family home, a large and light-filled house on a hill, not far from the centre of Enniskillen. Gordon was finding his feet in the business and Joan had resumed her career as a teacher. To the outside world they were a typically hard-working young couple, very much in love and with hardly a care. But they had already tasted the kind of tragedy that was to overshadow their lives. In June 1958, Richard, their second son, was born. He lived only two and a half hours.

Richard was born prematurely. Joan was so ill that she was not allowed to see him, and Gordon had to deal with everything. At two o'clock in the morning, summoned by a telephone call from Gordon, their minister arrived to baptise the little baby before he died. The grandparents were distraught. Joan remained in bed at the flat, where Richard had been born, and although Gordon was in deep shock, the arrangements for the funeral fell to him. He chose a small white coffin, and the grandfathers decreed that the baby should be buried in Joan's family graveyard at Tempo. Dazed the whole time and unable to be at her son's funeral, Joan recalls few details but remembers Gordon crying.

The trauma inflicted deep wounds. 'All that summer I could not bear to go near the graveyard, but after a few months Gordon took me there. We were out driving in the area, and he said, "Joan, I think you're ready to see where we laid the baby." So I went with him and looked at the little boy's grave. It was terrible. Even though this happened a long time ago, I still think about it and a feeling of great sadness comes over me at what might have been. I don't think that people ever get over the premature death of a baby. Gordon often talked about it, and all our children were told in due course about the death of baby Richard.' Joan still visits Richard's grave.

Peter was 23 months old by this time, and it was caring for him and watching his play and development that helped Joan to overcome her profound sense of loss. She realized that she had to pick herself up and give some support to Gordon, who was grieving as deeply as she was. It was this tragic experience which brought out a side of Gordon which she had not previously known. She felt his deep care for her, as well as his love. Despite his own grief, which he only expressed behind closed doors, he was a pillar of strength for Joan to lean on. She talked to her mother-in-law about her surprise at Gordon's depth of emotion. Granny Wilson told her that on the night Peter was born in a local nursing-home, having been phoned at 4.00 a.m. and told that he had a son, Gordon had gone to his room, where she could hear him crying with relief. He freely admitted to Joan later that he had 'cried like a child with relief and joy'.

When Marie died, the world thought that this was their first family tragedy, and when Peter was killed in a car crash, many people commiserated on the death of their only son. 'They were wrong,' says Joan. 'Our first tragedy was the death of Richard. I am convinced that it was the power of God which helped to pull me through, as it has done ever since, and certainly after the deaths of Marie, Peter and Gordon. When Richard died prematurely, I felt that God helped to slow me down, to take more rest, to take more care of myself, and to realize that life is so precious. When you are young you tend to take these things for granted . . .

The special relationship between father and daughter lies at the heart of the Gordon and Marie Wilson story. Though Gordon loved all his children deeply, there was a particular intimacy with Marie, perhaps because she was so open with him, and partly because she was the 'baby' of the family. And when she lay dying under the rubble of the explosion at Enniskillen, her last words burned an indelible impression on his heart, mind and soul. 'Daddy, I love you very much' were the last words he heard her say, and he carried them with him at all times afterwards—during his many radio and television interviews, during his numerous talks to groups both large and small in every corner of the British Isles and beyond, during his face-to-face meeting with the Provisional IRA, during his speeches in the Irish Senate and at the Forum For Peace and Reconciliation, during his meetings with the Queen, with President Mary Robinson, with political leaders in London, Dublin and elsewhere, and in private conversation with colleagues and friends. Those words, and all they meant, were the cornerstone of his philosophy and of his very life. They went with him to his grave, and yet they live on . . .

'The "bang" was the first thing I heard. The thought went through my head, "My God, that's a bomb going off!" But this was a sharp sound, sharp enough to tell me that the bomb was not at the far end of town but very close. I don't know how anybody else was responding at that moment, but I turned as I stood, and I managed to look over my right shoulder. Marie was on my right. I must have realized that the bomb had gone off behind me, and I remember seeing the wall beginning to crack up. This all happened in a split second, but it seemed at the time as if everything was happening in slow motion, like a television replay.

'Then it seemed to me that I was pushed forward, and I came down on my face. This must have been happening very fast, but at the time it didn't seem at all like that. It was like being pushed down on my face in slow motion; it was extraordinary, really. Certainly, it was all happening, or seemed to be happening, slowly enough to give me time to think yet again, "My God, we're in a bomb blast! But it can't be! Not here—not at the

Cenotaph on Remembrance Sunday!"

'At this point there was no sensation of noise that I can remember. There was no screaming, no shouting, but a kind of limitless, eerie silence. Having realized that the wall behind me was falling, I said to myself, "One big slab from that wall on top of you, boy, and that'll be the end—that'll be it—it'll be goodbye!" But when the wall had finally finished collapsing, there was only the sound of debris trickling down after it. And my mind flashed through the message to my spread-eagled body, "The big one didn't get you after all!"

'By that stage I was flat on my face, and I must have been pushed on my mouth and nose, because my glasses had come off. I realized that we were buried beneath several feet of rubble, but there was a chink of light coming through, and I could feel the rainwater on the stones. I thought that my glasses had been lost. Normally I can see very little without them, but in the middle of all that I was able to see sufficiently well to spot the glasses and somehow to put them back on again, with one hand. It seemed like a miracle at the time.

'With my glasses I could also see some blood trickling down a stone, and I knew then that I was cut. I had been taking an anticoagulent drug, and I was afraid that my blood would start to flow freely. As it happened, it was only a graze, and later the wound required only three or four stitches.

'All the time I was lying there on my mouth and nose, the noise level was increasing. Just after the blast there had been a sinister hush, a terrible quietness. And then the noise came, roaring and resounding and penetrating the several feet of rubble above us. There was shouting and moaning, and screaming, and yells of agony, until it all built up into a terrifying crescendo. At that stage a small voice inside me said, "I'm not too bad," and if that sounds like self-interest, it was also pure, basic human instinct, and a deep sense of thankfulness to be alive, even in a fix like that.'

In the midst of the blood, the hubbub and the screams of agony, Gordon's thoughts turned quickly to Marie. As they both lay under several feet of rubble, the events of the next few minutes were to inspire him, and also to haunt him, for the rest of his life:

'The explosion had thrown me forward, and my right arm was trapped. It later transpired that my shoulder had been dislocated, and therefore I had very little room for movement. At that point I realized that it was not possible to get out, certainly not without help from outside. But all through the screaming and shouting there was the urgent question in my mind: "Where's Marie? Is she hurt? Is she trapped? Is she alive?"

'Then, almost by magic, I found my hand being squeezed beneath that pile of rubble, and I knew it was Marie. She gripped my right hand and asked, "Is that you, Dad?" I could hardly believe that she was here, after all, lying beside me in the rubble. But the noise round about was increasing, so we had to shout louder and louder to make ourselves understood to each other. So we yelled, as best we could, amid the partial darkness and the noise.

'I shouted, "How are you, Marie?" She replied, "I'm fine." My heart skipped a beat with relief. But then, suddenly and terribly, she screamed. I knew that there must be something awfully wrong for her to scream like that. Again I asked her, "Are you all right?" And again came the reply, "Yes." But there seemed to be a bit of hesitation in that "Yes." A little later she shouted to me, "Dad, let's get out of here!" I replied, as best I could, "Marie, there's no getting out at the minute. We're trapped beneath all this rubble. But not to worry—they'll soon find us. There's a lot of people around, and they're certain to be digging down to us already. We've got enough air, there's a bit of light, and with God's help, we'll survive."

'But then she screamed again. I became desperately concerned about her condition. I could not, and I still cannot, understand how she could keep telling me that she was fine and yet, in between these messages of reassurance, she was screaming. Whether they were screams of pain or of terror I'll never know. I didn't know how badly she'd been hurt, but she was a very sensible girl of twenty, she had been trained as a nurse, and she would have known how to cope. She must have known she was hurt, and badly hurt. And I know now that she had been losing a great deal of blood by that stage.

'It must have been four or five times I shouted to Marie, "Are you all right?" But then, suddenly, her voice changed, and she sounded different. She held my hand tightly, and gripped me as hard as she could. She said, "Daddy, I love you very much." Those were her exact words to me, and those were the last words I ever heard her say. After that, her hand slipped away, and we lost touch.'

PART 3

A Windblown Spark

A Child That Didn't Live

for Dorothy and Don

*Though this poem is an elegy it had its origin in admiration—
admiration for the bravery and quiet bearing of our friends
as they went through the agonizing process of burying their tiny
child. The language of the poem is deliberately kept simple;
to mourn a dead child in words that are obscure or learned
(which of course may be fine in another context) seemed to be
almost defiling. The simplicity of the language is hopefully in
accord with the dead child's brief and uncluttered passage
through the world.*

So many came to the chapel in the maternity hospital
That we were standing packed together on the winding
staircase
Like refugees queuing in vain for a visa to a country
That didn't exist but yet we were trying to reach.

The death of an infant is a windblown spark too rapid to
be seen.
Life craves a span of light; we can only suffer so much
dark.
When you both came out of the morgue with that small
white coffin,
The size of a tradesman's toolbox or a weekend case

And placed it in the back seat of your car and got in
And drove off with it there behind you—your bravery
Drew all our love after you in the longest cortège,
Far beyond the high-walled cemetery and the tiny
unsealable tomb.

Elegy for a Still-Born Child

SEAMUS HEANEY

I

Your mother walks light as an empty creel
Unlearning the intimate nudge and pull

Your trussed-up weight of seed-flesh and bone-curd
Had insisted on. That evicted world

Contracts round its history, its scar.
Doomsday struck when your collapsed sphere

Extinguished itself in our atmosphere,
Your mother heavy with the lightness in her.

II

For six months you stayed cartographer
Charting my friend from husband towards father.

He guessed a globe behind your steady mound.
Then the pole fell, shooting star, into the ground.

III

On lonely journeys I think of it all,
Birth of death, exhumation for burial,

A wreath of small clothes, a memorial pram,
And parents reaching for a phantom limb.

I drive by remote control on this bare road
Under a drizzling sky, a circling rook,

Past mountain fields, full to the brim with cloud,
White waves riding home on a wintry lough.

Limbo

SEAMUS HEANEY

Fishermen at Ballyshannon
Netted an infant last night
Along with the salmon.
An illegitimate spawning,

A small one thrown back
To the waters. But I'm sure
As she stood in the shallows
Ducking him tenderly

Till the frozen knobs of her wrists
Were dead as the gravel,
He was a minnow with hooks
Tearing her open.

She waded in under
The sign of her cross.
He was hauled in with the fish.
Now limbo will be

A cold glitter of souls
Through some far briny zone.
Even Christ's palms, unhealed,
Smart and cannot fish there.

Gillin Na Leanbh

JOHN F. DEANE

Wife, child and I turned east from Dugort
strand, passed up by promontary forts
of the iron age, stood where sea-thrift
has worn the spiralling centuries, on a cliff

over the Atlantic; a patch of turf
lies sunk between field and cove on the damp edge
of nowhere. We stumbled on neglected, rough
slabs uninscribed and hidden now by sedge,

that mark where unbaptised were locked
in unblessed cells; misshapen, wailing things
half-born, hustled lives whom neither God
nor devil coveted, buried here when rings

of mist were beading round the moon; cachette
for pain, limbo, on the borders of being,
will any resurrection ever knit
life's proud continuum these children broke?

Not Just 'The Baby'

PATSY McGARRY

My grandfather Patsy McGarry is 33 years dead today. His was the first corpse I saw as he lay there on his bed. My nephew, Sam O'Connor, was three weeks dead last Friday. His was the last corpse I saw, as he lay there in his cot, his mother, father, grandparents, godparents, and all of us, standing around weeping.

My grandfather was 84, possibly 87—no one is sure. He was so old he could remember when Parnell died. Sam lived for just ten hours. He went from being a seemingly healthy nine pound ten ounce broth of a boy to his death with such speed, that no sooner were we aware of his arrival than we had to get used to the shock of his leaving. He had a rare blood disorder.

Despite a share of life's difficulties, we are a most fortunate family. We have not known too much of death. And though all of our grandparents have died, their passing was as it should be. It was in the order of things. No violation there. Our parents are very much with us, and we have always been healthy. As have our next generation.

So when my mother rang on the evening of Thursday June 12th to announce Sam's safe arrival, I heard the news with a certain nonchalance. When my sister Sinéad, Sam's aunt, rang at 2.30 a.m. the following morning to say he was very ill, I was jolted. When his father John rang at 5.30 a.m. to say he had died, I was stunned. And as the events of his passing unfolded, over the following hours and days, I began to realise that this ten-hour-old boy would leave a mark on all of us such as we had never experienced before. It ensures he will always be with us.

My sister Mary and her husband, John O'Connor, live at Ballykelly, near Cashel in Co. Tipperary. They have three other children, Róisín, Barney and JJ. Earlier this year when Róisín, who is four, became aware Mary was pregnant, she insisted the expected baby would be a girl. Her logic, as usual, was impeccable. God would not be 'so silly' as to send another one of 'them'.

Róisín has a strained relationship with her brothers. She even picked a name for her new sister. It would be Sarah.

As a precaution, and being more familiar with the silliness of God's ways, Mary and John asked her to choose a boy's name too. She chose Sam. And when Sam was born at the hospital in Clonmel, John rang home to break the news, gently, to Róisín. She took it very well. No doubt this was helped by the fact that Sam had brought presents with him for Róisín, Barney, and JJ. He brought Róisín a toy cat. She decided the cat was a girl, and called it Sarah instead.

A few hours later that evening staff at the local hospital became anxious about Sam, and he was sent to Ardkeen in Waterford. By the time he got there, he was seriously ill. John, who accompanied him to Waterford, realised he might not make it. He returned to Clonmel for Mary. By the time they got back, he was dead. Mary remembers he was still warm when she held him.

They brought him back to the hospital in Clonmel, where he lay in a cot next to Mary's bed for the following two days. She found it hard to part with him, and wanted all of us to see him first. So we would remember him, and as Sam, not just as 'the baby'. Lying there in his cot, he was perfect and still as a porcelain doll, his finely formed fingers interlaced. Strewn around him were a couple of stuffed toys and a small bouquet of three red roses from Ballykelly.

'He's dead,' announced Róisín, when she saw him. Then, examining him more closely she noticed how all his finger nails had darkened. 'Why are his nails painted?' she asked Mary, 'boys don't have their nails painted.' And Mary spoke to her about heaven.

Meanwhile, Sam's godparents, Seamus and Noelle Killeen, saw to the practicalities, while two other family friends, 'Aunty' Carmel and Rita, kept the show on the road as we and the O'Connors gathered and grieved. It is at such times you realise it's not such a bad old world that has such people in it.

My brother Declan drove my mother and sister there, instructing them forcefully en route that they were to keep a grip on themselves in front of Mary. But when all three arrived in the hospital room, it was he who was least prepared for the sight of Mary and Sam side by side.

The worst moment was on the Sunday morning, just prior to Sam's funeral. John took him to another room to be coffined, and Mary's heart shattered.

I had heard a mother ache like that just once before. It was in a graveyard in Dungannon, Co. Tyrone, in February 1993. Mrs Chris Statham watched as her only child, Julie, was lowered into the earth. Julie was twenty, and had taken her own life on February 2nd. The previous evening she had attended a month's mind Mass for her boyfriend, Diarmiud Sheils, and his father, Patrick, at their home near Dungannon.

They had been murdered by a UVF gang. They were just Catholics who loved Gaelic football and Irish music.

'It's so cruel,' wept Mary, as her son was taken away. And it is. Life is hard on mothers. They suffer in our coming and in our going. There were other bad moments. Mary being taken to the funeral in a wheelchair, still too weak to stand or walk. The sight of that small white coffin as it rested at an awkward angle on a trolley, inside a hospital exit. Seeing it lifted single-handed by an undertaker, and placed on the back seat of Mary and John's car. The small opening cut into a corner of the grave, where Sam would rest. Mary at the graveside in her wheelchair.

The funeral Mass was kept brief. What Mary and John needed, the priest said, was 'Christ's touch, not Christ's teaching,' and he urged us all to embrace and hug them. And we followed Sam to the small graveyard nearby, where he was buried with his grandfather, Bernard (Barney) O'Connor.

All of us returned to Ballykelly then, where we ruminated on the day's events as Róisín, Barney and JJ played to an attentive, unexpected, and large audience. Róisín kicked her cousin Garry in the shin, because he said her dog was stupid.

It was on the following day that the IRA murdered two young policemen in Lurgan. Leaving Rebecca (10), Louie (7), Abigail

(7), Joshua (3) and Katie (2), without a father. They were just Protestants who were seen as British symbols. It made me wonder once more whether anything is more unforgiveable than man-made grief. Or whether it can be forgiven at all. Sadness and sorrow. Bitterness too.

Lilies and Daffodils

in memory of Jenny, died February 1989, aged four

DAVOREN HANNA

During a period of great buoyancy in Davoren's life, he visited with his mother a circle of friends in the west of Ireland. While there he sparked up an intense relationship with a little girl called Jenny. A few months later Jenny died unexpectedly. Davoren wrote 'Lilies and Daffodils' for her parents and friends.

Bone-white —
she left prints
of her pale feet
upon wasted land.
Breathless she lay
at dove-dawn.

Why ruby the clouds
with your grief?
Look instead upon
her sunkissed daffodil
flaunting its yellow
death-defying head.

Child of Our Time

(forAengus)

EAVAN BOLAND

Yesterday I knew no lullaby
But you have taught me overnight to order
This song, which takes from your final cry
Its tune, from your unreasoned end its reason;
Its rhythm from the discord of your murder
Its motive from the fact you cannot listen.

We who should have known how to instruct
With rhymes for your waking, rhythms for your sleep,
Names for the animals you took to bed,
Tales to distract, legends to protect
Later an idiom for you to keep
And living, learn, must learn from you dead,

To make our broken images, rebuild
Themselves around your limbs, your broken
Image, find for your sake whose life our idle
Talk has cost, a new language. Child
Of our time, our times have robbed your cradle.
Sleep in a world your final sleep has woken.

17 May 1974

Not when you call them
do the pictures come

JASON SOMMER

In all of his alarm at the late departure
he still had his American thought for the day—
that he might be the only one in Ireland
at that moment who was concerned with time.
He retains the look of what he was doing:
fumbling the keys to the floor, slapping a book
under his arm—considering the lighted radio,
whether it needed extinguishing.
                                    Sometimes he left
it on for hours, a tree falling in the forest
and no one to hear. It might have been playing,
as it often did in his presence, great works
by the masters kept at bay in the background,
spending their largesse almost out of range,
but now it was saying a small country's news.
As he turned away to objects demanding sequence—
the bunched rug in the entry, the door, the lock—

the sounds at the verge of consciousness
became words as the ticking seems in motion toward us
in the dark bedroom, swelling into notice.
Perhaps it was just the syntax leaving till last
that the eight-year-old boy injured in the car
accident on the Naas Road, County Dublin,
in which his father had been killed, the child who was
expected to survive had died that day

which brought it in on him so, in past the simple
machine of his attention. So that he hardly
knew he had heard until he began to cry
for that son, and sat down to be late
for the class he was going to teach, feeling foolish
and yet instructed all over again, by force
as it seems he must be, in what he might have known.

Elegy for Mark

SHEILA O'HAGAN

*Mark died three days before his 21st birthday. He loved my
daughter and was a constant presence in my house. He was
thrown from his motorbike by a drunken driver. He died
instantly. In the instant before collision, he positioned his
motorbike downwards to save my daughter. I grieve for him
as for a son. He left behind a black coat he bought in Oxfam.
In the lapel he wore a silver rabbit pin.*

> In the stored past of an attic
> I, a woman growing old,
> Hold a coat, Oxfam with rabbit pin
> That shapes the lie of your presence,
> Arrange the sleeves in an embrace,
> Search for a familiar hair, a stain
> Mourning as older women do
> The bodies of the young,
>
>
> Watch how your shade invades the pool
> Of sun the window has let in,
> Hear the purr of the Silver Dream
> Racer along a country road,
> See it turn treacherous
> as you bend to the fatal spin,
> The reflection of your stillness

In the still turning wheels.

I, a woman growing old,
Perform a ritual for another's son
Loved as my own, rock myself
Into a grief black as the coat
I hold lest you be there, once a year
Climbing the height of this house
Far from any who might hear
The beat of the heart mending.

Áine

BERNARD O'DONOGHUE

In memory of Áine Murphy who died aged five months

*Áine was the daughter of my friends, Brian and Kathy Murphy,
two excellent Belfast musicians based in Oxford. Áine died
of 'cot death' as we were calling it then in 1993. The whole
local community here were heartbroken, Irish and English
alike; but the tragedy also became the occasion of hope—people
acting and mourning together in a way that was a symbol of
social healing. It was that positive feeling that stayed with us
in association with Áine's name, and that is what the poem
is trying to say.*

Those rosebuds I brought away
From the room in the crematorium
Where your small white coffin
Slid from view, wilted
On the car's plastic ledge
While we ate and drank, all of us,
Mourning your taking-off.
But two days later, look,
They're reaching up again
On a sunny windowsill,
Learning to stand
On stems, frail and graceful,
Pink bowls unbalanced
With perfect unease
On their long, green shoots.

Cot Death

DERRY O'SULLIVAN

For Willie, Teresa and family of Rangaroo, Bantry, Co. Cork

All we shared was absence
When they came to wake her
Late for the breast.
Her spilled-milk face
Curdled the blood.
Mouth to mouth the mother
Breathed into empty lungs
Useless as the dead smith's bellows
When exhaust choked the town.
Despair condensed in eyes
Searching the pocket-mirror
Pressed to her lips
For a smudge of moisture,
Only reflection, dry, pale, still.
My airmail breathless words
Could be scanned in vain
For moisture, flow, warmth,
While they waked her
And read the mass-cards,
As if I had caught death
Of that cold cot.

PART 4

That Was My First Death

Extract from Reading in the Dark

SEAMUS DEANE

Feet, September 1948

The plastic tablecloth hung so far down that I could only see their feet. But I could hear the noise and some of the talk, although I was so crunched up that I could make out very little of what they were saying. Besides, our collie dog, Smoky, was whimpering; every time he quivered under his fur, I became deaf to their words and alert to their noise.

Smoky had found me under the table when the room filled with feet, standing at all angles, and he sloped through them and came to huddle himself on me. He felt the dread too. Una. My younger sister, Una. She was going to die after they took her to the hospital. I could hear the clumping of the feet of the ambulance men as they tried to manoeuvre her on a stretcher down the stairs. They would have to lift it high over the banister; the turn was too narrow. I had seen the red handles of the stretcher when the glossy shoes of the ambulance men appeared in the centre of the room. One had been holding it, folded up, perpendicular, with the handles on the ground beside his shiny black shoes, which had a tiny redness in one toecap when he put the stretcher handles on to the linoleum. The lino itself was so polished that there were answering rednesses in it too, buried upside down under the surface. That morning, Una had been so hot that, pale and sweaty as she was, she had made me think of sunken fires like these. Her eyes shone with pain and pressure, inflated from the inside.

This was a new illness. I loved the names of the others—diphtheria, scarlet fever or scarlatina, rubella, polio, influenza; they made me think of Italian football players or racing drivers or opera singers. Each had its own smell, especially diphtheria: the disinfected sheets that hung over the bedroom doors billowed out their acrid fragrances in the draughts that chilled your ankles on the stairs. The mumps, which came after the diphtheria, wasn't frightening; it couldn't be: the word was funny and everybody's face was swollen and looked as if it had been in a terrific fight. But this was a new sickness. Meningitis. It was a word you had to bite on to say it. It had a fright and a hiss in it. When I said it I could feel Una's eyes widening all the time and getting lighter as if helium were pumping into them from her brain. They would burst, I thought, unless they could find a way of getting all that pure helium pain out.

They were at the bottom of the stairs. All the feet moved that way. I could see my mother's brothers were there. I recognised Uncle Manus's brown shoes: the heels were worn down and he was moving back and forward a little. Uncle Dan and Uncle Tom had identical shoes, heavy and rimed with mud and cement, because they had come from the building site in Creggan. Dan's were dirtier, though, because Tom was the foreman. But they weren't good shoes. Dan put one knee up on a chair. There was scaffold oil on his socks. He must have been dipping putlocks in oil. Once he had invited me to reach right into the bucket to find a lock that had slipped to the bottom and when I drew it out, black to the upper muscle, the slick oil swarmed down my skin to corrugate on my wrist. I sprinkled handfuls of sawdust on it, turning my arm into a bright oatmeal sleeve that darkened before Dan made me wash it off.

But it was my mother's and father's feet that I watched most. She was wearing low heels that needed mending, and her feet were always swollen so that even from there I could see the shoe leather embedded, vanishing from that angle, into her ankles. There was more scuffle and noise and her feet disappeared into the hallway, after the stretcher, and she was cough-crying as my father's workboots followed close behind her, huge, with the laces thonged round the back. Then everybody went out, and the room was empty.

Smoky shook under his fur and whimpered when I pushed him away. It was cold with all the doors open and the autumn air darkening. Una was going to die. She was only five, younger than me. I tried to imagine her not there. She would go to heaven, for sure. Wouldn't she miss us? What could you do in heaven, except smile? She had a great smile.

Everybody came in again. There wasn't much talking. My father stood near the table. I could smell the quayside on his dungarees, the aroma of horizons where ships grew to a speck and disappeared. Every day he went to work as an electrician's mate at the British Naval Base, I felt he was going out foreign, as we said about anyone who went abroad; and every day when he came back, I was relieved that he had changed his mind. Tom was pushing a spirit-level into a long leg-pocket of his American boiler-suit. Where would the little eye bubble of the spirit-level go now? Disappear into the wooden ends, go right off the little marked circle where it truly belonged? The circle would be big and empty. Dan picked up his coat, which had fallen off a chair on to the floor. I could see the dermatitis stains on his fingers and knuckles. He was allergic to the plaster he had to work with on the building site every day. Next month he'd be off work, his hands all scabs and sores. But Una would be long dead by then.

They all left except my parents. My father was at the table again. My mother was standing at the kitchen press, a couple of feet away, her shoes tight together, looking very small. She was still crying. My father's boots moved towards her until they were very close. He was saying something. Then he moved yet closer, almost stood on her shoes, which moved apart. One of his boots was between her feet. There was her shoe, then his boot, then her shoe, then his boot. I looked at Smoky, who licked my face. He was kissing her. She was still crying. Their feet shifted, and I thought she was going to fall, for one shoe came off the ground for a second. Then they steadied and just stood there. Everything was silent, and I scarcely breathed. Smoky crept out to sit at the fire.

That was my first death. When the priest tossed the first three shovelfuls of clay on to the coffin, the clattering sound seemed to ring all over the hillside graveyard, and my father's face moved sideways as if it had been struck. We were all lined up on the lip of the grave which was brown and narrow, so much so that the ropes they had looped through the coffin handles to lower it into the tight base came up stained with the dun earth. One of the gravediggers draped them over a headstone before he started pouring the great mound of clay in heaves and scrapes on top of the coffin. The clay came up to the brim, as though it were going to boil over. We subdued it with flowers and pressed our hands on it in farewell as we had pressed them on the glossy coffin top and on Una's waxen hands the night before at the wake, where one candle burned and no drink was taken. When we got back, the candle was out, and my mother was being comforted by aunts and neighbours who all wore the same serious and determined expression of compassion and sternness, so that even the handsome and the less-than-handsome all looked alike. The men doffed their caps and gazed into the distance. No one looked anyone else in the face, it seemed. The children appeared here and there, their faces at angles behind or between adults, fascinated, like angels staring into the light. I went up to the bedroom where Una had lain and sat on one bed and looked at hers and then buried my face in the pillow where her pain had been, wanting to cry and not crying, saying her name inside my head but not out loud, inhaling for something of her but only finding the scent of cotton, soap, of a life rinsed out and gone. When I heard noise on the stairs, I came out to see my uncles lifting the third bed from that downstairs room up over the banisters. They told me to stand aside as they worked it into the room and put it beside the bed where she had been sick. The wake bed was better; it had a headboard. Now Deirdre or Eilis would have one to herself.

Una came back only once, some weeks later, in early October. My mother had asked me to visit the grave and put flowers on it. They would have to be wild flowers, since shop flowers were too expensive. I forgot until it was almost four o'clock and getting dark. I ran to the graveyard, hoping it would not be shut. But it was too late, the gates were padlocked. I cut up the lane alongside the east wall until I reached the corner where the wall had collapsed about two feet from the top. It was easy to climb over, and inside there was an untended area where the grass was long and where I had seen flowers growing before. But there was not a one, not even on the stunted hedgerow beneath the wall— not a berry, not a husk. I pulled some long grass and tried to plait it, but it was too wet and slippery. I threw the long stems away into the air that was already mottled with darkness, and they fell apart as they disappeared. Running between the little pathways that separated the graves, I got lost several times before I found the fresh grave and recognised the withered flowers as those we had left a short time before. I pulled the wreaths apart, hoping to find some flowers not so badly withered, but there were very few. A torn rose, a chrysanthemum as tightly closed as a nut, some irises that were merely damp stalks with a tinge of blue—that was all. But I couldn't get them to hold together with the bits of wire from the original wreaths, so I scooped at the ground and put them in a bunch together, pressing the earth round them with my foot. All the while, I was saying her name over and over. Una, Una, Una, Una, Una. It was dark, and I felt contrite and lonely, fearful as well. 'I have to go,' I said to the ground. 'I have to go. I don't like leaving you, but I have to go, Una.' The wall seemed far away. I got up off my knees and rubbed my hands on my socks. 'I'll come back soon.' I set off at a run, along the dark pathways, zig-zagging round headstones and great glass bells of airless flowers, Celtic crosses, raised statues, lonely, bare plots, another even fresher grave, where the flowers still had some colour even in the shrivelled light that made the trees come closer. She, it was Una, was coming right down the path before me for an instant, dressed in her usual tartan skirt and jumper, her hair tied in ribbons, her smile sweeter than ever. Even as I said her name, she wasn't there, and I was running on, saying her name again, frightened now, until I reached the wall and looked back from the broken top stones over the gloomy hillside and its heavy burden of dead. Then I ran again until I reached the street lamps on the Lone Moor Road, and scraped the mud off my shoes against the kerb and brushed what I could of it from my clothes. I walked home slowly. I was late, but being a bit later did not matter now. I didn't know if I would tell or not; that depended on what I was asked. I knew it would upset my mother, but, then again, it might console her to think Una was still about, although I wished she wasn't wandering around that graveyard on her own.

My older brother, Liam, settled the issue for me. I met him in the street and told him instantly. At first he was amused, but he got angry when I wondered aloud if I should tell my mother.

'Are you out of your head, or what? You'd drive her mad. She's out of her mind anyway, sending you for flowers this time o' year. Sure any half-sane person would have said yes and done nothing. Anyway, you saw nothing. You say nothing. You're not safe to leave alone.'

All night, I lay thinking of her and hearing again the long wail of agony from my mother halfway through the family rosary. It made everybody stand up and Smoky crawl back under the table. I wished I could go in there with him but we all just stood there as she cried and pulled her hair and almost fought my father's consoling arms away. All her features were so stretched. I hardly recognised her. It was like standing in the wind at night, listening to her. She cried all night. Every so often, I would hear her wail, so desolate it seemed distant, and I thought of Una in the graveyard, standing under all those towering stone crosses, her ribbons red.

Stillborn

(with acknowledgements to Matthew, aged 6)

SIOBHÁN PARKINSON

These were my son Matthew's actual words, several months after his brother Daniel was stillborn, on hearing adults using the term 'stillborn' and suddenly realising precisely what it meant.

'Oh! Is *that* what it means?' he said.
'I thought it meant
He was still born
Even though he was dead.'

There are Three People in Heaven

MAIRÉAD CAREW

dedicated to Fiach McDonald, aged four

*My baby daughter, Órfhlaith McDonald, died on 2 January
1996 in a cot death, aged seven months. Fiach was three and
a half years old at the time.*

'There are three people in Heaven,'
he explained.
'My granddad, Michael,
my uncle Tommy
and my little sister, Órfhlaith.

Órfhlaith grows taller.
She plays with Winnie the Pooh,
and she still shakes her rattle.

Tommy and Michael let her play snap
even though she's only small
and Uncle Tommy wins all the games
because he cheats.'

Nuair a ba Ghnách liom Luí le mo Thuismitheoirí

CATHAL Ó SEARCAIGH

Bhíodh mo thuismitheoirí ag iarraidh codladh
nuair a déarfainn leo i dtólamh
go raibh an leabaidh faoi dhraíocht
is go raibh sí ag imeacht de rúide reatha trasna na
  spéire;
is ar ócáidí den chineál seo
bhíodh réaltóg ag spréacharnaigh leo
fríd fhuinneog an tseomra leapa;
a gcara sa chosmos
a dtreoraí fríd an dorchadas.
'Joe,' a déarfainn leo—
mo dheartháirín a fuair bás
is a bhí ansiúd ar an uaigneas;
ach tharraingeodh siad an t-éadach amach thar a
  gceann
is thiontódh siad a ndroim liom
lena bpleidhce beag ainglí, lena bpáistín fionn . . .

dalta an tseandomhain spíonta seo
a chaitheas faoiseamh a fháil fosta ón tsolas róbheo.

When I Used to Sleep with My Parents

CATHAL Ó SEARCAIGH

Translated by Anna Ní Dhomhnaill

My parents would be wanting to sleep
When I would always say to them
That the bed was bewitched
And that it was making a mad dash across the sky,
and on occasions like this
a star would be winking at them
through the bedroom window:
their friend in the cosmos
guiding them through the darkness.
'Joe', I would say to them—
my little brother who had died
and who was there in the loneliness:
but they would draw the clothes around their heads
and they would turn their backs to me
their roguish little angel, their happy little child . . .

just like this tired old world
which must also seek respite from the overactive light.

Mid-Term Break

SEAMUS HEANEY

This poem was written about ten years after the events it recalls. One thing it does not record is what my father said to me (as the eldest child) on the morning of the funeral. 'Don't be crying. If you cry, they'll all cry.' But I think we all did, anyhow.

I sat all morning in the college sick bay
Counting bells knelling classes to a close.
At two o'clock our neighbours drove me home.

In the porch I met my father crying—
He had always taken funerals in his stride—
And Big Jim Evans saying it was a hard blow.

The baby cooed and laughed and rocked the pram
When I came in, and I was embarrassed
By old men standing up to shake my hand

And tell me they were 'sorry for my trouble',
Whispers informed strangers I was the eldest,
Away at school, as my mother held my hand

In hers and coughed out angry tearless sighs.
At ten o'clock the ambulance arrived
With the corpse, stanched and bandaged by the nurses.

Next morning I went up into the room. Snowdrops
And candles soothed the bedside; I saw him
For the first time in six weeks. Paler now,

Wearing a poppy bruise on his left temple,
He lay in the four foot box as in his cot.
No gaudy scars, the bumper knocked him clear.

A four foot box, a foot for every year.

For Edward Hartnett

born October twelfth, 1942
died November twenty-ninth, 1942

MICHAEL HARTNETT

My brother Edward died in 1942, a baby. I was one year old.
I do not remember him, of course, but he was often mentioned
by my parents.

1
birds cross
the lunar apex
and cry down
the saltmade balconies of stone:
his voice from bill of seamew,
caved in his limbo,
Edward.
that I should mourn, he speaks
out of the earth he has become,
his sound
the echo of his longing to be here.
every gathering of branch and cliff
star and wingclip
calls him here,
implies his absence:
I have borrowed his life
and perhaps, his poetry.

2
we are alone:
toned by rock
the wind gesticulates
and white by moon
the sea throws up its arms.
we are alone
because the dead are alone.

Lucy's Song

CATHERINE PHIL MacCARTHY

This poem is dedicated to Lucy Partington who was murdered in 1973, aged twenty-one years.

Uncover my bones, long dead and clean,
The moon of my skull that gleams in the mire,
Hold me to your breast, carry me unseen.

From this vile place, where I have been
Dismembered for years, a brutal lair,
Uncover my bones, long-dead and clean.

Blood of my blood, this is no time to keen,
Work by colour of the dawn air.
Hold me to your breast, carry me unseen.

From the mouth of hell, unthread my spine,
Ribcage, pelvis, sacrum, in order,
Uncover my bones, long-dead and clean.

From a chest of oak, let goodness shine,
a jar of honey, music of a choir,
Hold me to your breast, carry me unseen,

Sister my sister, your love is mine,
I move with you, the silence is clear,
Uncover my bones, long-dead and clean,
Hold me to your breast, carry me unseen.

Marbhghin 1943: Glaoch ar Liombó

(do Nuala McCarthy)

DERRY O'SULLIVAN

Saolaíodh id bhás thú
is cóiríodh do ghéaga gorma
ar chróchar beo do mháthar
sreang an imleacáin slán eadraibh
amhail líne ghutháin as ord.
Dúirt an sagart go rabhais ródhéanach
don uisce baiste rónaofa
a d'éirigh i Loch Bó Finne
is a ghlanadh fíréin Bheanntraí.
Gearradh uaithi thú
is filleadh thú gan ní
i bpáipéar *Réalt an Deiscirt*
cinnlínte faoin gCogadh Domhanda le do bhéal.
Deineadh comhrainn duit de bhosca oráistí
is mar *requiem* d'éist do mháthair
le casúireacht amuigh sa phasáiste
is an bhanaltra á rá léi
go raghfá gan stró go Liombó.
Amach as Ospidéal na Trócaire
d'iompair an garraíodóir faoina ascaill thú
I dtafann gadhar de shochraid
go gort neantógach
ar a dtugtar fós an Coiníneach.

Is ann a cuireadh thú
gan phaidir, gan chloch, gan chrois
i bpoll éadoimhin i dteannta
míle marbhghin gan ainm
gan de chuairteoirí chugat ach na madraí
ocracha.

Inniu, daichead bliain níos faide anall,
léas i *Réalt an Deiscirt*
nach gcreideann diagairí a thuilleadh
gur ann do Liombó.
Ach geallaimse duit, a dheartháirín
nach bhfaca éinne dath do shúl,
nach gcreidfead choíche iontu arís:
tá Liombó ann chomh cinnte is atá Loch Bó
    Finne
agus is ann ó shin a mhaireann do mháthair,
a smaointe amhail neantóga á dó
gach nuachtán ina leabhar urnaí,
ag éisteacht le leanaí neamhnite
i dtafann tráthnóna na madraí.

Stillborn 1943: A Call to Limbo

(for Nuala McCarthy)

DERRY O'SULLIVAN

Translated by Michael Hartnett

*I grew up as the eldest of 11 children (or so my parents led me
to believe). After my father's death in 1980, my mother re-
vealed to me the existence of a stillborn, unnamed brother
buried in unconsecrated ground where graves of such children
were unmarked and which had been a famine pit, apparently.
Nuala McCarthy, a Bantry mother, refusing to hide her own
loss, has fought since the '60s for a public recognition of this
spot as a sacred monument. The burial details were authen-
ticated by my mother before she died.*

You were born dead
And your blue limbs were arranged
On your mother's live bier—
Umbilical cord still intact,
An out-of-order telephone line.
The priest said you were too late
For the blessed baptismal water
Which flowed from Milky Way Lake
To anoint the faithful of Bantry.
You were cut from her
And folded unwashed
In a copy of the *Southern Star*,
World War headlines pressed to your lips.
They made a coffin for you from an orangebox
And your mother listened to the requiem
Hammering in the corridor
As the nurses assured her
That you were a dead cert for Limbo.
Out the gate of the Mercy Hospital
The gardener carried you under one arm—

A funeral of dogs barked with you
All the way to a patch of nettles
Called the Rabbit Warren.

There you were buried
Without prayer nor stone nor cross
In a shallow hole alongside
A thousand other stillborn babies—
The hungry dogs waited.
Today, forty years later,
I read in the *Southern Star*
That theologians no longer
Believe in Limbo.
But believe me, little brother,
Whose pupil never saw the light,
When I say to Hell with them all:
Limbo exists as certainly as Milky Way Lake
And it's there your mother lives,
Her thoughts burning her like nettles,
Every newspaper a prayer book
As she listens for unwashed babies
In the evening bark of dogs.

PART 5

An Inextricable Love

Birth Mother

CATHERINE PHIL MacCARTHY

That Christmas she asked for
photographs. Without parents.

I checked the last roll of film
developed, feeling her eyes

smart along a sleeve
all the way to a tiny fist.
That first glimpse,

risked over hot whiskey
in the quiet of a bar
at closing-time,
silken brown hair
slipping over

an inextricable love
the wide river of her breath

sparkled with red leaves,
intertwined limbs,

her heart breaking
all over again
in the white turmoil
of rapids.

Birth Certificates

EVELYN CONLON

At the time of giving birth a mother is prone to the most extraordinary feelings, not all of them tinged with carefree forgiveness. I had the experience of being in the bed next to a woman like this woman and years later, when writing this story, realised that she was the person I remembered most clearly from that lying-in experience, as it is hilariously called.

The woman today wondered what life was like now for the woman who had been in the bed beside her.

'I remember she told me that she was an alcoholic. I said that she couldn't be, not at nineteen, but then the visitors came from AA so she must have been. She said she never remembered getting pregnant—maybe she did but couldn't admit it. She was giving the baby up. Up to where? I used to think as we both lay, trying not to disturb our stitches. "They say if I keep it I'll only go back on the drink." "Who are they?" "The friends from AA and my mother" (who had come sneakily on her own, supposedly going for a check on her varicose veins, and never looked at the child once). "They say! They say! But what do you say, Linda, what do you say?" "Well, I know one thing, I'm not taking it out of that basket. It's not fair to expect me to do anything with it. I'm giving it up, amn't I? The nurses can change its nappy." And I began to feel privileged to wash the shit from around my baby's bottom. I put my nipple into my baby's mouth, touching his cheek with it first so he snuggled his mouth round and open, burying his nose in my breast.

'My baby drank guilt, as I could see from the corner of my eye Linda's basket untouched, writhing instead of rocking between the bedposts where it was hung, sending screeches up and up, its mother with stone for a face, and then a nurse would come. "Now Linda," she would say, "you know it's best if you get to know it. Then you won't feel later that you had no choice." "I'm not touching that basket." And there I was, allowed to feed my baby with my very own nipple because I could take it home because a man had asked me to marry him and I had said yes, or maybe I had asked him. Think of anything, I whispered to my baby as inconspicuously as I could manage. When Linda left the ward I always picked him up and squeezed him properly and then I would go to Linda's basket where I would lay my fingers on her child's head and say some tight useless cliché.

'Forty-eight hours after Linda and I had pushed our babies out, I turned on my left side and saw her move towards her basket. She leaned up on her hunkers, then thought better of it, moved again, then back. There was a god playing with her to see how much magnet she was. She got down from the bed carefully and pulled herself ghostlike to the basket. She dug her hands into it, clenching her eyes, and came out with a baby. She seemed surprised at it, then kissed it full on the mouth. I heard her whisper as if the words were escaping from her. So from then on my baby drank tears and apprehension because Linda would not leave her baby out of her arms even when the nurses said, "Come on now, it needs to sleep; come on, you need to sleep." "I can sleep all I like later," she said.

'I asked to be let out a few hours early because I hadn't the stomach to watch the passing over of Linda's baby to an intermediary, who would then pass it over to some married infertile couple. That's how I came to leave the hospital on a Sunday morning instead of a Sunday evening.'

Extract from Stolen Child

BAIRBRE NÍ CHAOIMH AND YVONNE QUINN

Stolen Child is based on the true story of a woman's search for her natural mother. The mother herself had been brought up in an industrial school by an enclosed order of nuns. In 1952, at the age of twenty-three, she became pregnant and gave birth to a baby girl in a Dublin maternity hospital. However, as an unmarried mother there was no question of her being allowed to keep the child and it was immediately put up for adoption. She did not see her daughter again for forty-three years.

It was a girl. They handed her to me and she was like a flower with its petals fluttering in the wind. Like a tiny bag of bones. I held out my finger and her own fingers closed round it. At last I have someone of my own, I thought. The nurse looked at me funny. 'Let's put her in the cot over here,' she said. 'You don't want to go spoiling her.'

'I'm calling her Rose,' I tell the other women. 'After my Mammy.' At night I wake up with me chest aching and just look at her. None of the other mothers love their baby half as much. The doctor walks down the ward like an emperor. All the other men in white coats come after, half bowing. They stop at us. Maybe to say how well you're looking. 'Not married,' he says, in that uppity voice. My face burns. I lie down then and when I wake up you're gone. Cot and everything. I close my eyes and open them again but you're still gone. It's like Mother Benedict and the *Irish Roses*. One day she brought a box in and let us all take two. Then she made us put them back again. 'You didn't think I was going to let you keep them,' she said. Ha ha ha. And she belted herself and laughed again.

'They took your baby,' the woman in the next bed whispered. 'That doctor came back for her. About an hour ago.' I run shouting up and down the ward. 'Give her back to me. Give me my baby back.' 'You never had a baby. It's your imagination,' they say. 'And sure even if you had itself, you're not married, how could you look after it?' 'Give her back to me.' 'You'll have to leave now,' they say.

It's a grand sunny day outside. As if nothing had happened. I walk and walk and feel very tired. Scouring the place for you and your soft blonde head. My breasts leak and the blue milk runs in rivers down my front. It's like the rain sometimes. You don't notice it and then you're sopping.

'Why are you crying?' this man says. 'There's a convent round the corner. Why don't you go there? The nuns will help you.' 'Go to hell,' I tell him.

The Pomegranate

EAVAN BOLAND

The only legend I have ever loved is
the story of a daughter lost in hell.
And found and rescued there.
Love and blackmail are the gist of it.
Ceres and Persephone the names.
And the best thing about the legend is
I can enter it anywhere. And have.
As a child in exile in
a city of fogs and strange consonants,
I read it first and at first I was
an exiled child in the crackling dusk of
the underworld, the stars blighted. Later
I walked out in a summer twilight
searching for my daughter at bed-time.
When she came running I was ready
to make any bargain to keep her.
I carried her back past whitebeams
and wasps and honey-scented buddleias.
But I was Ceres then and I knew
winter was in store for every leaf
on every tree on that road.
Was inescapable for each one we passed.
And for me.
                            It is winter
and the stars are hidden.
I climb the stairs and stand where I can see
my child asleep beside her teen magazines,
her can of Coke, her plate of uncut fruit.
The pomegranate! How did I forget it?
She could have come home and been safe
and ended the story and all

our heart-broken searching but she reached
out a hand and plucked a pomegranate.
She put out her hand and pulled down
the French sound for apple and
the noise of stone and the proof
that even in the place of death,
at the heart of legend, in the midst
of rocks full of unshed tears
ready to be diamonds by the time
the story was told, a child can be
hungry. I could warn her. There is still a chance.
The rain is cold. The road is flint-coloured.
The suburb has cars and cable television.
The veiled stars are above ground.
It is another world. But what else
can a mother give her daughter but such
beautiful rifts in time?
If I defer the grief I will diminish the gift.
The legend will be hers as well as mine.
She will enter it. As I have.
She will wake up. She will hold
the papery flushed skin in her hand.
And to her lips. I will say nothing.

Extract from The Love Test

HUGO HAMILTON

After six months in detention at Hohenschönhausen, Christa became more heavy and slow with her pregnancy. The hysterical panic of the first months had given way to a dull boredom of the spirit. She became more detached and tranquil, floating on the intimate companionship with the baby inside her. The baby's movements placed her in a half-dream, like a constant anaesthetic.

She had cried all she could. She had no idea what had happened to Ralf. She knew only one thing, that she would wait for him through all of this, as though she possessed that primitive faculty of supreme patience which made it possible to continue through the loneliness and banality of time. Pregnancy made her immune to the taunts of the female wardens, to the degrading strip searches.

Every morning at 5 the door of her cell was flung open and she was led down the corridor towards the kitchen. Her walk was slow, almost regal. How often had she counted the neon lights and the diamond shapes of the lino, and the pattern of doors unlocking and relocking behind her all the way to where she reached the sudden reek of fat and stale soup in the kitchen? How often had she prepared the same *Eintopf,* every day, every week?

The long hours spent standing were excruciating on her spine. She still sometimes cried convulsively, not knowing how long she would be in prison. Once or twice she had thought of killing herself and the baby. But then, as the months passed, the baby became her only salvation.

She had more than once been informed by Pückler that there was going to be a trial, but it never seemed to come. Nobody, not even the doctor, had said anything as yet about the baby's future, except some of the other female workers in the kitchen who told her the baby would be taken from her. 'You won't even see it,' they said.

She worried about Ralf. Pückler had said nothing about him except to make a sign with his index finger across his throat. Christa refused to believe it and sensed that he was alive in the same prison, perhaps only a few hundred metres away in another wing. Preparing the plates each morning she placed one extra piece of bread on one tray. Each midday she placed one extra lump of meat or an extra dumpling in one bowl, keeping Ralf alive in her thoughts, even though she understood the outrageous odds required for it to reach him.

She suffered heartburn. At night she dreamed of milk and apples. And escape. At times she began to see love as an escape. If her sortie to West Berlin with Ralf had been an attempt to elude destiny, then her imprisonment too, like her pregnancy, seemed to her a natural consequence of having loved too much. She regretted that she had not rejoiced more while freedom was so abundant. Life in prison reflected all the uncertainties of illness. It brought with it the same false hopes she had so often seen as a nurse in the eyes of patients, as though the whole prison institution were a disease: the walls, the grey steel doors, the threadbare blankets and the worn lino in the kitchen.

For a few days before the trial Christa was taken out into the sun for two hours a day. Though she didn't know it, it was to improve her colour, to make the accused appear as though she had been treated well. The trial itself was over almost before it even began. She was brought by van to the court. She had been offered her civilian clothes, though none of them fitted her, except the shoes. The court room was small, with red velvet curtains on the windows and a portrait of Lenin on one wall. The court was full of Stasi personnel. Behind a desk sat two men in plain clothes.

Ralf appeared through a door on the far side of the court. Their eyes met, not with any sense of affection or hope but with a mutual recognition of deep, intractable fear. It was a look that haunted her long afterwards. He seemed older, more gaunt, though his face too was brown from the sun. He was handcuffed and made to sit down behind a desk on the other side of the room, surrounded by guards carrying submachine-guns. She kept looking at him, hoping to receive some sign. But he was in a dream, not even listening when the charges were read out. Pückler handed a statement to the magistrate. Ralf was asked about the Zeiss money. He denied the charges and said nothing more.

Christa wanted to show Ralf some sign of her loyalty, and when she was asked by the magistrate about the money she stood up, allowing Ralf to see how pregnant she was, until she was pushed instantly back into her seat again.

The judge sentenced Ralf to fifteen years in Hohenschönhausen. Ralf seemed unmoved as he was led away towards the door. Then he stopped and looked back at her. 'Tell them about us, Christa . . .' he shouted. Then he was roughly pushed out through the door and, though she heard him shouting in the corridor, she couldn't make out what he was saying. She heard the magistrate sentence her to three years and recoiled at the shock. Her child would be almost going to school by then, she thought, bursting into tears.

Days later she gave birth. For once the guards were more understanding when she could no longer work in the kitchen. For once they didn't shout and the doctor was summoned to take a look at her. The midwife came and administered an injection. The handcuffs looked idiotic over the rounded arch of her stomach as she was taken from her cell, and all the time, as the baby was kicking, she wondered if all the fear in this environment would have an effect on it.

The familiar smells of the hospital came to Christa as a great sense of safety. She tried to speak to the nurses and find solidarity in their profession, but a warden standing by the bed ordered her to be silent. The midwife listened to her stomach as Christa looked at the woman's face, at the grey hair underneath the nursing cap and the gentle, reassuring hands around her tummy. She put all her trust in this silent authority.

Within hours she began to go into labour. Even then Christa wanted to keep the baby inside her, as though giving birth were like giving the baby away, like losing everything she had with Ralf. The midwife began to give instructions in a forceful voice, commanding her to push, and it didn't take long before Christa heard the baby crying out, a sweet lungful of air claiming a place for itself in the world.

Christa blacked out, and when she came round again the midwife was standing beside her.

'I'm sorry,' she said. 'We tried everything we could.'

'What do you mean?' Christa said.

'I'm so sorry, it was stillborn, my dear.'

Christa sat up. Even her physical exhaustion could not keep her down. 'It can't be true. That's a lie,' she said. 'I heard the baby cry just now . . .'

'Now come on, *Liebchen*. Don't upset yourself,' the midwife said, hovering around her with grotesque kindness.

The Year 1912

translated by Eoghan Ó Tuairisc

—The trunk.

She said the word offhand yet there was a touch of stubbornness in her tone. She hadn't agreed to go to Brightcity with her daughter a week ago last Saturday to buy the trunk, and it irked her like a white frost the way it had been perched up on the ledge of the kitchen dresser, adored like an idol. The children having great play with it, opening it, closing it, looking it all over. She hadn't the heart to vex her daughter this final week, otherwise she would have cleared it off into the room under the bed. But tonight, though the daughter might be of a different mind and anxious to show off that expensive article to the company that had gathered, the mother had followed her own inclination of nightfall and moved the trunk into the room—it might, she said, get damaged or scratched where it was.

It was like a burnt spot or a smallpox scar on the face of life, tonight especially since she seldom had a hearty gathering under her roof. It was useful and wellmade, but that was only a chimaera, a ghost from the Otherworld come to snatch away the first conception of her womb and the spring of her daily life, just when the drinking, the high spirits, the music and merrymaking were in full spate. Seven weeks ago, before the passage-money came, she had been as much on edge awaiting it as Máirín was. That her daughter should be off to America was no surprise to her, no more than the eight sisters of her own whose going was a bitter memory still. She had been schooled by the iron necessities of life to keep a grip on her feelings and throttle her motherlove—as Eve ought to have throttled the serpent of Knowledge. It was the passage-money that had set the heather ablaze again. Flickers of affection, flashes of insight from shut-away feelings, were setting her sense and reason aglow with the knowledge that this going into exile was worse than the spoiling of a church or the wreck of a countryside . . .

But it was destiny, must be attended to. The day was agreed. Patch Thomáis was gone for the sidecar. Back in the crowded kitchen the merriment had risen to a frenzy; remnants of the wreck of a people, doomed to extinction at daybreak, bringing their ritual vigil to a hurried night's-end climax of wild debauch . . .

A halfpenny candle stood on a small press by the wall in the bedroom, smeared by a breeze coming by the edge of the paper on a broken windowpane. Depth, magic, mystery of unfathomable seas, reflected by the guttering candleflame in the trunk's brass knobs. It was of pale yellow timber, the mother couldn't at once remember where she had seen that colour before—the face of a corpse after a long wake in sultry weather. And a certain distaste kept her from looking into the trunk, that same tabu which had kept her, though she had often tried, from looking at a corpse in a coffin.

—Have you everything? she asked the daughter keeping her eyes off the dimlit thing. There were all kinds of things in it—a sod of turf, a chip off the hearthstone, tresses of hair, a bunch of shamrock though it was autumn, stockings of homespun, a handful of dulse, items of clothing, papers connected with the voyage across. The daughter took her shoes, coat, hat and dress out of the trunk and laid them on the little press to put on her. During the week she had often laid them out like that but the mother had never encouraged her, and early in the night she had implored her not to put them on till morning.

The mother shut the trunk, threw the bedquilt over it. —To keep it clean. She had long feared that the daughter once she was in the American clothes would be estranged from her, alien as the trunk. Máirín was in her stocking feet and naked except for a long white shift which she had been at great pains to fix about herself that evening and which she had no intention of taking off until she had reached the house of a relative on the other side. Seeing her like that was to see a vision, the only one which had remained clearskinned and beautiful in her memory. A vision that gave bodily shape to the dear lost Tree of Life, while it made real the delicate and deceitful skin of the Knowledge-Apple—a mother's first conception, first fruit. She had so many things on the tip of her tongue to say to her, the intimacies, the affectionate things saved up in motherlove, her lifestuff, from the moment she feels the quick seed in her womb until the flush of eternity puts out the twilight of the world.

For a month now she had said many things to the daughter, scraps scattered at long intervals . . . that she couldn't care if all in the house were to go so long as Máirín stayed . . . that the whole house would miss her, herself especially . . . that of all her children she was the one who had given her the least trouble . . . that she was fine about a house. But none of all that said what she wanted to say. She felt like a servingwoman, the necklace she was putting about the young queen's neck had broken, its precious stones scattered here and there in danger of being crushed and broken. She felt as if some hostile force were filtering her speech, hindering her from letting loose the flow of talk that would ease the tight grip on her heart. She was aware she could never hope to express the things in her mind in a letter which she would have to depend on someone else to write, and in a language whose make and meaning were as unhomely to her as the make and meaning of the Ghost from the Fairymound. And a letter was a poor substitute for the living contact of speech, eyes, features. Her flowing imagination, floodtide of her love, would run thin and freeze in a niggardly writing.

She was hardly likely to see her daughter again for a very long time. Máirín would have to repay her passage, then earn the passage of one or two more of the family, as well as send a share home. It could happen that the child in her womb would set eyes on her before she did. That American coat, the graveclothes—how tell one from the other? The 'God speed her' that would be said from now on had for its undermeaning 'God have mercy on her soul'. Children often got those two expressions mixed up. And when the time came that in actual fact would change the 'God speed' into 'God have mercy', it would come without a decent laying-out and a bier to be carried, and with no passionate keen. Even the graveclothes, no mother would have them awhile to shake out the folds of them from time to time as a relief to her anguish, and there would be neither name nor surname on a rough bit of board in the churchyard by the Fiord for generations to come. The voyage—that immensity, cold and sterile—would erase the name from the genealogy of the race. She would go as the wildgeese go.

But while such ideas were as a sour curd in the mother's mind, she wouldn't give in to the thought that she would never see the daughter again. Her sense and reason said no, her love, hope, determination, said yes. And it was these she listened to. Yet even if she were to see her again she knew she'd be utterly unlike the simple country girl, now nineteen years old, with a look pure as morningsun on a hillside in the Promised Land. Her lips would have been embittered by the berries from the Tree of Good and Evil. That dark weasel envy in her heart. Experience, that slimy serpent, writhing in her mind. Temper of cold steel in her countenance. The tone of her voice transformed by the spell of a harsh stepmother. Such were all returned Americans. She must reveal herself to her now, as the mother of warriors in the cave used to reveal herself to her children when every sally-ing out in search of food was a matter of life and death. Reveal herself to her while her age and ignorance were still unmocked at, while there was yet no wall of disbelief between her daughter's mind and hers . . .

The money, she thought, was the best way to begin. She took a cloth purse from her bosom, took out what small change the daughter might need in Brightcity, and gave her the purse with the rest. The daughter hung it about her neck and settled it carefully in her breast under her holy scapular.

—Look now child you take good care of it. It's likely you won't need it at all, but if you fail to find work soon it would be too much to be depending on Aunt Nora who has her own children to look after. Keep the rug tucked well round you on the vessel.

Make free with no one unless it happens to be someone you know. You'll be safe as soon as you reach Nora's house. Even if you have to take small pay, don't overstrain yourself working . . . You will make a visit home after five years. Well, at least after ten years . . . It can't be but you'll have a few pence put by by then. My . . .

She had kept her spirits nicely up to that. But as soon as she thought to break the crust of speech she couldn't find a word to say but stood stockstill staring at her daughter. Hands fiddling with the folds of her apron. Blushing, tears and smiles painfully together in her cheek. Humps and wrinkles of distress coming in her forehead like keys struggling with a lock. The daughter was almost dressed by now and asked where was the small change she'd need in Brightcity? The mother had been so eager to talk that she had forgotten to get a little purse to put it in. Turning to get it she fell into such confusion she forgot the money in her fist until it fell and scattered about the floor. Her idea had been to wait till her tongue could contrive a proper speech, then to hand over the small change to the daughter as a sacred offering, embrace and kiss her . . . Instead, the sacrifice had been ripped from her hand.

Putting away the little purse the daughter felt an envelope in her pocket. —A tress of your hair, mama, she said. I thought I had put it in the trunk along with—the rest. She held the black tress between her and the candle, her blue eyes softened, became childlike. She felt an urge to say something to her mother, she didn't quite know what. Her thoughts went fumbling here and there as a stranger might among the blind holes of a bog on a dark night. The pair of them would have to be in the one bed, the light out, and a wand of moonlight through the small window to charm and set free the tongue. She looked her mother in the eyes to see if she might find encouragement there, but she remained unconscious of her mother's seething emotions, locked within, quite unable to crack the fixed and rigid mask of her features.

She put on the light and gaudy coat, then the wide-brimmed

hat. Part of the preparations for her attack on life, she supposed, was to spend a long time fixing and refixing the set of the hat, though she had no idea which particular slant she wanted. She didn't realise that the size and the undulations of the hatbrim added nothing to her good looks, nor that the yellow shoes, black hat and red coat made a devil's own trinity in conflict with her fresh and delicate features. But she was ready: hat, coat, low shoes on and lady-gloves—not to be taken off again. She felt strange, surprised as a butterfly that feels for the first time that it has shed its cramped caterpillar limbs and has the endless airy spaces unimpeded to sail through on easy wings. She felt too some of the lightheaded pride of the butterfly . . .

The mother forgot until the trunk had been locked that she had forgotten to put a bit of hendirt in it, or somewhere among the daughter's clothing. But she wouldn't for the world unlock it again. She couldn't bear the daughter to make fun of her, this morning especially, accuse her of pishrogues and superstition. She shook a tint of holy water on her, and while she was putting the feather back in the bottle the daughter was off out to the kitchen floor to show off her American ensemble.

The sidecar hadn't come yet. There was a swirl of dancing. Tom Neile with his back to the closed door was singing *The Three Sons* in a drunken voice drowning the music—

There's many a fine spa-a-rk young and hea-a-rty
Went over the wa-a-ter and ne-e-e-r return'd.

—Tone yourself down, said the mother to Tom, but she'd have given a deal just then to have a tune like he had in order to release the load of her love in a spilling song. The girls had gathered again about the daughter, scrutinising her rigout, although they had been a week looking at it. They gave the mother no chance of keeping her company. They thought nothing, it seemed to her, of driving a wedge into nature, one almost as inhuman as that driven in by the immense cold sterile sea. The young women were chirruping of America. Chirruping of the life they'd have together soon in South Boston. Typical of a race whose guardian angel was the American trunk, whose guiding star was the exile ship, whose Red Sea was the Atlantic. Bidín Johnny reminded her to ask her cousin to hurry with the passage-money. Judeen Sheáin told her on her life not to forget to tell Liam Pheige about the fun there was at the wake of old Cáit Thaidhg.

—Take care you don't forget to tell our Seán that we have the Mountain Garth under potatoes again this year, said Sorcha Pháidín. He said when he was going that after him no one would ever again be born to the race that would attempt to sow it, it was such a hardship.

—Tell my boy, Máirín, that it won't be long till I'll be over to him, Nora Phádraig Mhurcha said in a whisper that all the girls heard.

—By cripes it won't be long till I'm knocking sparks out of the paving stones of South Boston myself, said a redhead youth whose tongue had been loosed by the drink.

—God help those that have to stay at home, said old Séamas Ó Curráin.

The whiskey was circling again. —Here now, you ought to take a taste of it, said Peaitsín Shiubháine who was measuring it out, heeling the glass towards Máirín with a trembling hand. He splashed some of it on her coat. —A mouthful of it will do you no harm. Devil the drop of poteen you're likely to see for the rest of your life. There was an undertone to his voice, he was remembering the five daughters of his own who were 'beyond'— one of them thirtyfive years gone—and he had no hope of ever seeing them again . . . I'll drink it myself then. Your health, Máirín, and God bring you safe to journey's end.

Neither Peaitsín nor anyone else in the gather thought to add, —God send you safe home again. Such ignorance of the proper thing to say sparked off the mother's repressed anger. —Five years from today you'll see her back home again, she said tartly.

—God grant it, said Peaitsín and Seáinín Thomáis Choilm together.

—And she'll marry a monied man and stay here with us for good, laughed Citín, Máirín's aunt.

—I'll have little or nothing to show after five years, said Máirín. But maybe you'd marry me yourself, Seáinín, without a sixpence?

But by this time Seáinín had huddled himself back against the door and was talking like a tornado to let the mockery of the young girls pass over him.

—At all costs don't pick up an accent, said a young lad, one of her cousins, —and don't be 'guessing' all round you like Micilín Éamoinn who spent only two months beyond and came home across the fields with nothing to show for his voyage but half a guinea and a new waistcoat.

—Nor asking 'what's that, mamma?' when you see the pig.

—Anyhow, you'll send me my passage, said Máiréad the next daughter to Máirín, eyes sparkling.

—And mine too, said Nóirín the next sister.

The mother felt a bleak touch of her own death hearing the greedy begging voices of the pair. Years of delay were being heaped on her daughter's return, as shovelfuls of earth are heaped on a coffin. And the grace of that homecoming was receding from her—as far as Judgement Day. At that moment the children she had given birth to were her greatest enemies.

She set Máirín to drink tea again though she had just stood up from it. But she wanted to come close to her again. She must break bread, make a farewell communion, weave the intimate bond of a farewell supper with her daughter. She would tell her plain and straight that she didn't believe this parting meal to be a funeral meal as far as home was concerned: there would be an Easter to come, before the Judgement. But they weren't left to themselves. Her sister Citín with her family of daughters and some of the other girls pushed up to the table by the wall and in no time had Máirín engulfed among them.

The daughter had no wish for food. Her face burned: desire, panic, wonder, an anguish of mind, all showed in her cheek. Brightcity was the farthest from home she had ever been, but she had been nurtured on American lore from infancy. South Boston, Norwood, Butte, Montana, Minnesota, California, plucked chords in her imagination more distinctly than did

Dublin, Belfast, Wexford, or even places only a few miles out on the Plain beyond Brightcity. Life and her ideas of it had been shaped and defined by the fame of America, the wealth of America, the amusements of America, the agonised longing to go to America . . . And though she was lonesome now at leaving home it was a lonesomeness shot through and through with hope, delight, wonder. At last she was on the threshold of the Fairy Palace . . . Tremendous seas, masts and yardarms, blazing lights, silvertoned streets, dark people whose skin gleamed like beetles, distorting for her already the outlines of garth, mountain, rock, fiord. Her mind tonight was nothing but a ragbag to keep the castoff shreds of memory in until she might shed them as flotsam as she sailed. She was so unguarded now that she let herself be led out to dance on the stone floor, dressed as she was for America. In any case she couldn't have found it in her heart to refuse Pádraigín Pháidín.

It irked her conscience that she had so long neglected him. She began to dance in a lackadaisical way, but the pulse of the music—that music to which they were beholden even in the fairyplace—excited an impulse in herself, and soon in her dappled outfit she was like a young alien deer, fullblooded, with the common young animals of the herd prancing about her, inciting her to show what she was made of, what she could do, while the elders sat around in sage contemplation. The mother was thinking that if she was ever to see her again the hard experience of life would then be a dead weight on that lust for dancing. In place of that passion of young and eager blood that wedded her limbs to the graceful movement of the stars, the thin and watery stuff of greying age would be keeping her tired bones fixed on earth.

Nevertheless the mother was closely watching, not the daughter, but Pádraigín Pháidín who was dancing with her. There and then she guessed the whole story. Easy to see. Very likely the pair had never said a word of love to each other. Very likely they hadn't said a word tonight. And they were likely never to say a word in their lives. But she realised they would be married in

South Boston in a year's time, in five years, ten years even . . .
She was vexed. That's what lay behind Pádraigín's wild dancing
fit. What she had failed to say in words he was saying in dance.
Body and limbs he was enacting a perfect poem, with growing
zest, abandon, vigour and precision, until a lash of his nailed
boot carved a spark out of the hearthstone in time with the final
beat of the music. Some might put it down to intoxication, but
the mother knew better. That spark was in fact a finishing touch,
a final fling of the spirit in full victory. Then hardly waiting to
be asked while still breathless from the dance he began with
easy power to sing. And the mother forgot the daughter listen-
ing to him:

> The garden's a desert, dear heart, and lonesome I be,
> No fruit on the bough, no flower on the thorn, no leaf,
> No harping is heard and no bird sings in the tree
> Since the love of my heart, white branch, went to Cashel
>   O'Neill.

A young spirit trying to crack the shell of a universe that shut
it in, so fierce was his song. By now the mother had come to
hate him. An evil being, fingering her own proper treasure . . .
Horse's hooves and the clatter of a sidecar were heard from the
cart-track outside. Music and merriment ceased suddenly. Only
Seáinín Tolan stretched drunk against the shut door still moan-
ing—

> Ora, wora, wora,
> It's on the southern side of New York quay
> That I myself will land—

the only snatch of a song Seáinín ever raised.

—Indeed you'd be a nice gift to America! Devil drown and
extinguish you, it's a pity it isn't on some quay you are, a useless
hulk, instead of here, cried a youth who could stand him no
longer.

The trunk was taken from the room and set like a golden calf
on the table.

—Take out that and tie it up on the sidecar, said the mother.

—It might get broken, said Máirín. Leave it alone until I'm ready to go out along with it. That trunk was her licence and authority to wear an elegant hat on her head and an ostentatious coat on her back instead of a shawl. Without the trunk her lady-outfit would be an insult to God. If she let it out of her sight for as much as a second as like as not those tricksome and showy garments would wither into rags and ashes about her body.

She turned now to say goodbye to those who hadn't the strength to accompany her as far as the king's highway. Crippled oldtimers who could barely manage to shuffle across the street; for most of them this was likely the last time they'd leave their own firesides for a social occasion. This was the first link of the chain to be jerked apart, it made her feel for the first time how hard the parting was, how merciless. Whatever about the rest of the people, she would never set eyes on those again. In spite of her distress and hurry she looked closely at each one of them so as to store up in her memory their shape and features. She kept a grip on her emotion and broke down only when she came to her grandmother at the hearth. She had as much affection for her grandmother as she had for her mother, and made more free with her. And was loved in return. Never a week went by but the old woman had laid aside a bit of her pension to give her, whatever else might be behindhand. The old creature was as speechless as if already turned to clay. In fact she almost was, for the best part of her was in the grip of 'the One with the thin hard foot', and the rest waiting on busy death to prepare her dwelling-place. Her mouth was as dry as the timber of a new-shut coffin, and except for a faint blinking of the eyelids that brought her far-off look a little closer to the here and now, Máirín would have thought that she hadn't the least notion what was going on.

—I'll never see you again, mammo, she said, her voice breaking at last in tears.

—God is good, said the mother, a shade stubborn.

Then to kiss the small children and the infant in the cradle. She felt it as a warm substantial summer after the midwinter chill. Charming her senses against the threat of the graveclothes.

The mother brought her off to the room once more. But they weren't long there till Citín and Máiréad came in on them to get their shawls so as to accompany Máirín to Brightcity. The mother could have melted them. How officious they were— without them, she thought, the lump of sorrow in her throat wouldn't have hardened again. All she could say to Máirín was that she'd have good earnings; that she hoped they'd have good weather at sea; and for the life of her not to forget to have her picture taken beyond and send it home.

—My own darling girl, she said picking a speck of fluff from the shoulder of the coat and giving a hurried quirk to the hatbrim, though the daughter at once reset it her own way. And having glanced quickly round the house she was ready to go.

The sidecar went lurching down the rugged village track followed by a dense crowd, men, women and children. They had all the appearance of a sacrificial procession: the sidecar like a funeral pyre ahead, puffs of the men's tobacco-smoke hanging in the early morning air, and Máirín walking in her barbaric costume as the officiating druid.

The mother walked alongside the daughter and offered to carry her rug, but Bríd Shéamais snatched it and carried it herself. She had determined to have Máirín under her own wing on this last walk, but Citín and her own Máiréad thwarted her once more. Then all the young girls closed round her, some chattering and laughing, some so lonesome at her going that they hadn't the heart to say much, and others sorry that they weren't in her place or going along with her. By this time the mother had hardly any feelings of regret left so angry was she with the rabble that wished to deprive her of her daughter before she was even out of sight. She took a spleen against the sidecar too. It was moving as fast as if it was giving a corpse 'the quick trot to the graveyard'. It seemed to her that it was the trunk—perked up on the box of the car, its timber blond as an ear of corn in the rays of the virgin sun—that was picking the horse to death's own scything speed. She hadn't a word left to say . . .

There was a mild red light from the sun just up. Field walls and piles of stone grinned bleakly. In the little pokes of fields slanting and rugged the tramped stubble was like the head of some Samson having suffered the shears of Delilah. A small sailingboat just out from harbour with a fair wind scratched a bright wake down the Fiord. Máirín looked back from the rise at Hollycliff, from then on her own house and the village houses strung around would be out of sight. Last year's new thatch joined the old black and withered roof at the ridge-strip—line of contact between the past and the time to come. And the village seemed asleep again after its brief second of action, slight as a spit in the ocean that the sailingboat might obliterate.

The sidecar halted at the end of the track. The people formed a close group in the mouth of the highway so that the mother was cut off from the daughter. Just another stray stone in the cairn, that's all she was. The same as if she was neither kith nor kin. More than ever she begrudged Citín and Máiréad their going to Brightcity with Máirín. When the kissing began the women were like a gaggle of scavengers about a prey. They pushed their way rudely up to her daughter, squeezed her hand, snatched kisses one after the other like a flock of starlings on a trash-heap. The men shook hands with her, shy, laconic, seeming to say it was all one, and if it had to be done then it were best done as quickly as might be. Pádraigín Pháidín did likewise, but unlike the rest of the men he gave the slightest lift to his head and the mother caught the eyes of the couple interlocked for the nick of a second.

At last it was her turn. She hadn't kissed her daughter since she was a child. But she failed to put much yearning and anguish into the kiss, though her lips hungered for her. Hadn't she kissed all and everyone? Hadn't all and everyone got ahead of herself in the kissing and hugging? The daughter's kiss was cold and insipid, the good skimmed from it by all that had been pecking at her. Her body was cold too, cold and insubstantial as a changeling from the Liss.

But what quite spoiled the kiss for her was the sight of the trunk, she was unable to keep her eyes off it and it was all but whispering in her ear—

No mortal kiss will break the spell of the changeling, seduced by pleasure to wander and forget, whose dwelling is the golden web which young desires weave from the sunlight on green hills far off from the here and now.

Máirín was now on the sidecar. Máiréad sitting beside her, Citín next to the driver on the other side, Pádraigín Pháidín fixing the trunk firmly between them up on the box. Damned spirits, they appeared to the mother—the accursed trunk, Máiréad greedy to get her passage-money, and Pádraigín Pháidín on edge to get to America and marry her daughter—three damned spirits torturing her first-born and best-loved.

Pádraigín had finished and the people were moving aside to make way for the horse. The women started in to sob, and the sobbing lifted into a loud wail of words, expressing no real anguish the mother thought, beyond voice and tears. They wouldn't leave her even the comfort of keening alone. And she shed no tear . . .

She stammered uncertainly, —I'll see you before five years are out. And couldn't raise her eyes to meet the eyes of her daughter, not if the sky fell.

The car was now moving. Sobbing the daughter whimpered, —You will. But now the mother's heart as well as her commonsense knew that she would not. Pádraigín Pháidín would see her sooner and the girls of the village and her own children, even the infant then in her womb. The mother realised she was but the first of the nestlings in flight to the land of summer and joy: the wildgoose that would never again come back to its native ledge.

PART6

The Year the Spring Didn't Come

A Childless Woman

KERRY HARDIE

With young women I am motherly,
with older women, daughterly,
with women of my own age, lonely.

1
First a landscape smudged with sound
and trickles of sound.
Air threaded with rain.

Where the swollen river has loosed its brown waters
into the marsh-places
and the shine of the cold sky shows in flatness of
flood—
there the frogs grunt,

heave, flop about in watery eruptions,
stilling when they hear us,
but for an old bull, quivering, out of his head with
sex,
who regards us balefully from his station
on a female, mostly submerged
in the spawny glub and not protesting.

It is all woven—woods, sounds, light;
before the frills and flutterings begin.

2
I have a part-time, not-mine, son,
loaned from a woman that I never meet.

Sometimes I wonder if she thinks of me.

3
It's no big deal, happens over and over.
Just haunted, in spring, by the slow file
of the grey women who have made me.
And I am them, and I am breaking the line.
This is what it means: the year the spring didn't
come.
Spilled water, seeping underground.

A fragile time, February going into March.

4
I am become a woman standing on the sidelines,
on station platforms meeting and seeing off trains,
casually surprised to be remembering
with gifts the anniversaries of friends' children.
A woman given
to speaking carefully, saying mostly the generous
thing,
watching the brown flow of rivers,
waiting by windows open to the dusk.

Childless

JANET SHEPPERSON

Slinky, screeching, dark, they skite about
like swifts in next door's garden, following
their flightpaths through an airspace that can turn
solid for them to slide on, hang from, swing—

or wanting the sound of the waves, they redesign
their strip of grass and bushes as an island,
they prance into the spray and scurry back,
bedraggled, damp, to catch hold of her hand.

'Mummy, he says I'm ugly.' 'He says I'm a girn.'
'Well then don't play with him. There's other fish
in the sea.' The kitchen window is a lighthouse,
from far out in their boat they see it flash

as they tack unsteadily across the garden,
then the real rain starts. I hear her call them in.
I watch the walls of their house bulge and turn liquid
with laughter, till the rooms rock up and down.

Our house is childless. Rooms have never stretched
nor walls dissolved. These mornings we sleep long
in a bed engulfed by sand. Each month we carve
fantastic shapes and wait for the tide's tongue

to snake up the moat and lick the sides till they
crumble
under the sea's huge swirling swishing run,
hemming us in and dragging us out and crowding us
to the edges of our lives. But it never comes.

Because of the sea's absence we hear the wind
louder and louder all night, becoming the voice
of absence itself, commenting on the dull
parade of space after space after space after space.

The Famine Road

EAVAN BOLAND

'Idle as trout in light Colonel Jones
these Irish, give them no coins at all; their bones
need toil, their characters no less.' Trevelyan's
seal blooded the deal table. The Relief
Committee deliberated: 'Might it be safe,
Colonel, to give them roads, roads to force
from nowhere, going nowhere of course?'

one out of every ten and then
another third of those again
women—in a case like yours.

Sick, directionless they worked fork, stick
were iron years away; after all could
they not blood their knuckles on rock, suck
April hailstones for water and for food?
Why for that, cunning as housewives, each eyed—
as if at a corner butcher—the other's buttock.

anything may have caused it, spores,
a childhood accident; one sees
day after day these mysteries.

Dusk: they will work tomorrow without him.
They know it and walk clear. He has become
a typhoid pariah, his blood tainted, although
he shares it with some there. No more than snow
attends its own flakes where they settle
and melt, will they pray by his death rattle.

You never will, never you know
but take it well woman, grow
your garden, keep house, good-bye.

'It has gone better than we expected, Lord
Trevelyan, sedition, idleness, cured
in one; from parish to parish, field to field;
the wretches work till they are quite worn,
then fester by their work; we match the corn
to the ships in peace. This Tuesday I saw bones
out of my carriage window. Your servant Jones.'

Barren, never to know the load
of his child in you, what is your body
now if not a famine road?

Exorcism

CATHERINE PHIL MacCARTHY

Nothing prepared me for
the change in your voice.
The story of how

you buried her little girl,
surrendering to the grave
in the small coffin

your own birthless years.
April swept rain from the headland
and ditches inclined

whitethorn buds
and not a soul knew
your dreams were

chrysanths scattered
from your hands
on the raised earth.

Extract from Mother of Pearl

MARY MORRISSY

*Mother of Pearl is a novel about mothering. This extract
explores the idea that we all nurture a dream of a child
(perhaps merely a version of ourselves as children) and can
imagine that child into existence.*

Deferentially they both withdrew; sometimes in the night Stanley
would reach out for her tentatively, a flutter across her breast.
But if Irene felt the blushing smart of her own desire she would
damp it down. She had wished to be united in pleasure, not to
be observed in it. The act of being looked at, at being done to,
was weighed down with memories of Granitefield. She remem-
bered the men she had saved. Their wanting, their yawning long-
ing had always seemed to Irene more precious than the consum-
mation which had expressed itself only as desolate relief, their
moment of abandonment as functional as expectorating into the
sputum jug beside their beds. She was glad that Stanley would
never achieve this, the lonely spilling of seed and its death-like
aftermath, the terrible spentness of it. It kept him apart from
them; it made of him someone proud and unassailable, one who
had secrets of his own he was not willing to share. She did not
resent this. Rather, she fed on other tendernesses which Stanley
offered, often unknowingly. His hand on the nape of the neck,
the soft, burly strength of his embrace, his worshipping gaze.
She loved the geography of his face, a country she had explored
with her fingertips and the rough crevices of his blameless hands.
She liked to watch him shave, the fluffy application of soap, the
delicate dabbing of the shaving brush, the dangerous scrape of
the cutthroat, his skilful mastery of jaw and cheekbone. When
they went to church—she still did not believe but she went for
his sake—she liked to link him on the street. It made her feel
anchored, his bulk beside her steady and reassuring, a bulwark
against the resistance she felt all around her.

She would always be a stranger here; the very street seemed to exhale disapproval. A brooding sense of violence seemed to seep from the bricks; at night she imagined she heard the pounding of troops on the slimy cobbles, the crashing down of doors, the seizure of captives in the dark. Stanley chided her; it was all in her head, he said. The neighbours hailed Stanley merrily when they were together but when Irene ventured out on her own she felt reproof and wariness in their greetings. She knew what they wanted from her—information, some means of placing her. A family name they could trace, a townland however distant they could ascribe to her. She was an unknown quantity among them and she knew that the only way she could counter that was to bear a child, whom they could claim as one of their own. The first thing they asked if they met her at the dairy or in the church porch was 'Any news?' By that, they meant one thing, the one thing Irene knew she could not deliver.

'Why do they torment us like this?' she would ask Stanley.

'They're just concerned, that's all.'

'They're just nosy, that's what you mean. Don't know how to mind their own business. Why can't they just let us be?'

Stanley would shrug and turn away. But as time went by he too began to dread the dogged enquiries after Irene's health. He would dodge neighbours on the street if he saw them first, longing for the simplicity of those years alone with his mother, a union without any expectations.

But away from their prying glances, Irene's presence, the very fact of her gave him courage. When she was not there he fell prey to a sense of foreboding, convinced she would not come back. If she travelled to the southside of the city, he imagined a catastrophe; a train crash; a murder. He felt oppressed in the backwash of her departures, surveying the cluttered house to reassure himself. She could not bear empty spaces. She had filled the rooms with all sorts of trinketry. Decorative plates adorned the walls, spotted delph sat proudly on the dresser. She had pinned pictures from magazines and cut-outs from greeting cards on the walls of the kitchen. Old calendars showing Alpine scenes still hung though their dates no longer had a bearing. She collected ashtrays, though neither of them smoked, souvenirs of places she had never been. Brighton, Inverness, St Helier. There was one without a declared place of origin, a gruesome object, molten-like, as if it had been boiled down from ghoulish droppings or lava. Greetings from Mount Etna, Stanley thought wickedly. She crocheted covers for things, cushions, tea cosies, even a pouch for the lavatory paper, as if everything must be disguised or dressed up as something else. The neighbours, he knew, considered the decor fanciful and further evidence of Irene's oddness. But he liked the busyness of it. It was like living in the stall of a bazaar; who knew what treasures lay hidden here? It was in this way he felt Irene had made herself known to him, substitutes for the small worries, the female confidences he had expected. Instead, she offered her delights—the antimacassars, the doilies, the paper blossoms—with a girlish flourish. Their significance was lost on Stanley. Guiltily, he mistook them as shows of gratitude.

In years to come both Stanley and Irene, separated by distance and circumstance, would look back on the early years of their marriage as a surrogate childhood, a time on which the adult world had made no claim. He would recall the sense of protection she inspired in him, the telling gestures that indicated anxieties she would never speak of. He noticed how she examined her arms, fingering spots or exploring her wrist or elbows as if for bruises or marks of some kind. He felt she was looking for traces of illness, her old illness. She was conscious of the scar left by her operation and would always undress in the dark as if someone, other than him, was watching and would be shocked, though by then it was no more than a red seam on her flesh, like a light scrape with death.

Irene, in turn, would remember Stanley's softness, which in the harsh light of Granitefield she had determined as weakness but which she came to recognise as a kind of helpless power. She marvelled at what he allowed her to see of him, his fearfulness, his resigned acceptance of the world, even the absence of desire. It seemed to her that all of these should have been hidden; for Irene what kept people intact was what they withheld. Her father, Dr Clemens—though she never considered them in the one breath—were understandable, one for his brutality, the other for his professional kindness, because by their nature they had achieved a safe, knowable distance. But Stanley occupied a place dangerously close to her; he entrusted her with knowledge she felt she shouldn't have. She worried that she might use it against him.

He was afraid of moths, she discovered. She came upon him in the bedroom one night, standing as if transfixed, while a moth flapped helplessly near the light bulb. He was stripped to the waist like a man about to do battle and it was only when she noticed his fingers clenched white around the collar of his shirt that she realised his terror. The moth was trapped behind the parchment shade. Its frantic clatter, the frenzied movements of a creature so small—it was inconceivable to Irene that this could be something to be afraid of. She was tempted to mock but something stopped her, some delicacy of the moment. She whipped the curtains closed and switched the light off. The mesmerising whirring ceased with the swift plunge into darkness, but Stanley still stood paralysed. She could sense the throb of his fear across the room.

'It's still in here somewhere,' he said. 'I can't sleep knowing it's here.'

So Irene would spend many daylight hours hunting away sleeping moths. How clever they were, she thought, melting grainily into wood, inhabiting the darkness and making it their own. Only the light fooled them; they threw themselves at it and betrayed themselves.

It was a hazy morning in April when Irene met Martha Alyward outside the Monument Dairy on the corner of the street. Irene had always considered her a rival. A flaxen-haired woman born in the same year, the mother of three school-going sons. She had the knack of delicately prying into other people's lives. For Irene she was the epitome of Jericho Street—neat, tight-lipped, right-eous. She fastened on to gloom, grimly watchful for the worst. An accident in the shipyard, a sick child, a drowning in the river. News of these invariably came through Martha who fed needily on the awfulness of the world.

'And how are we today?' Martha asked setting down two bulging bags of shopping. She took Irene in in one swift, critical glance. Irene had lost count of the number of times she had been surveyed in this fashion followed by the same sly enquiries and for Irene the inevitable humiliation of not being able to offer even the smallest of prizes. The pre-ordained pattern of it depressed Irene. She usually tried to avoid engaging Martha in conversation but sometimes, like now, it wasn't possible. She longed to be able to silence Martha, to shock her into submission, to get the better of her. The thought of such a victory made her suddenly giddy.

'I'm not the best, to tell you truth,' she offered cryptically.

'Oh?' prompted Martha.

Irene watched her expression change. A greedy curiosity replaced her usual pitying concern. Irene could not bear it. She pounced.

'I've been feeling queasy these past few mornings . . .'

'Oh?' Martha repeated.

Irene could smell blood; she was surprised at how easy it was. Martha needed only the vaguest implication.

'At first I thought I'd eaten something that disagreed with me. You know the way it is, you never think about the obvious . . .'

It was a moment of pure spite.

'You're not . . . ?'

Irene glorified in Martha's dumbfounded surprise. After four years, even she had stopped asking 'Any news?'

'Well,' Martha said finally, 'and when are you due?'

'November,' Irene said triumphantly.

'You'll have it in the Royal, I suppose?'

'Oh no,' Irene replied, moving away, 'I'll be going south.'

Stanley was the last to hear. Len Alyward stopped him on the street as he trudged home after the evening shift. He waved heartily from the bald patch that counted as his garden. He grew roses. Stanley was always amazed that anything would grow in the soot-laden air. Secateurs in hand, Len wandered across the street.

'Well, aren't you the boyo?' He laid a hand on Stanley's shoulder.

Stanley looked at him blankly.

'I knew you had it in you!' He nudged Stanley in the ribs. 'Oh come on, Stan, the whole street knows. You know what Martha's like. Bush telegraph!'

Len snapped the secateurs playfully. 'Congrats, old man, the first of many, eh?' He shook Stanley's hand. 'A celebration is in order, don't you think?'

Stanley frowned, still trying to figure it out. Len had always had the capacity to make him feel dull-witted.

'Give over, man, don't be coy! It isn't every day a man finds out he's going to be a father!'

From that moment, Stanley believed. Out of the mouth of Len Alyward, here on the dusty, weathered street, it just had to be true. They went to the Crown. Gold and gleam and the pour of liquor, ale that seemed to have taken on the colour of wood. The raucous jollity of the place—the crones in the snug, the scrums of dockers—convinced him that the whole world was in on the secret. The noises of their revelry danced in his fogged brain. He drank to prolong the moment of belief. After years of grounded loyalty, he felt the joy of the convert. The world had taken wings. He was no longer a rocky outcrop; he was joined, hip and heart. And Irene had made it possible, somehow.

It was two in the morning by the time he made it home. Irene, awake and fearful, heard his key in the lock. He fumbled with it several times before slotting it into place. He leaned heavily against the door after shutting it. Irene heard the pause as a gathering up of rage. She had seen it many times with her father, like the pawing of a bull before the charge. Her sense of victory over Martha had long since dissipated, giving way to a bleak panic. This lie, the calculated misunderstanding she had set in motion, would undo them both. It would strip everything bare. It would make visible the void at the centre of their marriage. And all the other deceptions would become obvious too. Stanley would know what she had become at Granitefield and would see it as Davy Bly had done, as a piece of whoring. She had thought of fleeing—she got as far as rescuing her suitcase from the attic—until she realised there was nowhere to go, and no man to save her.

She lay in bed listening to Stanley's heavy tread on the stairs, strangely exhilarated by the imminence of danger. When they were first together she had longed to be bruised by him, to have blue mottled marks on her thighs, love bites on her neck. A black eye, even. He entered the room, and sat heavily with his back turned to her on the other side of the bed.

'I met Len Alyward,' he offered, an explanation for his condition and the lateness of the hour.

Irene braced herself. She stretched out a hand to touch him. It was a conciliatory gesture but she fully expected the swipe of his fist in return. Instead he turned to her, his features blurred by drink bathed in an expression of almost beatific gratitude.

'I'm going to be a father,' he said.

It was Stanley who gave the child a name. It will be a girl, he declared with proud certainty, and she shall be called Pearl. Pearl had been his mother's second name, he explained, the one she had favoured herself. He was like a man bewitched, intoxicated with unexpected passion. So this, he thought, was what Rose Toper had felt when she would declare mournfully 'I love you'. It wasn't like walking on air, as she had said, it was like being air. He was in flight, a glorious, airy sensation. From his lofty height everything seemed steeped in munificence. The house, the street, the ghastly, jagged outlines of the city had become benign, withdrawing like respectful elders allowing them to luxuriate in their new-found joy. Even Irene seemed transformed. There was a curious grace in her movements now; he could see her thin, hard body, roundening and softening, and her watchful gravity becoming serene.

The new devotion Stanley lavished on her was the care Irene associated with a mother. It was the kind of love Stanley knew all about. He stopped her carrying coal in from the yard. He made her take naps in the afternoons. He worried extravagantly about her health. He would help her rise from the low armchair in the parlour, placing his hand in the small of her back. In the evenings he came home with shop-bought cake. Basking in this new solicitude, she felt prized and cosseted as if she were a delicate, doomed child. To watch him during those months was to know what he would have been like had he been in love with her. His tenderness bloomed into something active and joyful, their marriage—for her, an escape, for him a need for shelter and protection—had become a right and fitting union. The child she had conjured up out of light and air had done all of this. Like a fairy or a sprite (no earthly child could have done it) she had waved a wand and granted them a wish. Irene wondered when he would call a halt to the make-believe while secretly hoping it would last just a little while longer, if only to delay the punishment she knew would inevitably come. And yet, in the midst of it, Irene imagined she could feel a stirring in her womb as if a little being was sprouting wings in there. Stanley would press his hand to her belly and believed that he felt something too. Between them they had formed a child destined to be lost. A pearl of great price.

It didn't last, of course, Stanley's flight. After three months of dizzying dislocation he fell to earth. It happened at the entrance to the shipyard. A light drizzle was falling. Summer seemed to have retreated behind a thicket of grey cloud. There was a large crash, the thump and boom of a girder falling to the ground from a crane that had been stealthily moving across his line of vision. A siren started wailing and there was the crunch of boots on gravel as men rushed to the scene. Matthew Earley, they cried, it's Matthew! Stanley stood, rooted to the spot. Above him the arm of the crane hung like the limb of a deformed god. The gaping belly of a liner with men crawling like insects over it, the agonised cries of the wounded one . . . and the spell broke. It was not Matthew Earley who lay pinned beneath a lump of iron, it was the coiled form of an infant, whom Stanley had been carrying for months. She disintegrated before his eyes, her smooth, glazed face like the remnants of eggshell trampled in the dirt. He stooped to pick a fragment up, something to remember her by, but there was nothing on the ground but tiny shards of glass and the stink in his nostrils of his own foolishness.

The miscarriage was announced at the beginning of the fourth month. (Irene had spoken of it too soon, the neighbours said quietly among themselves; she had tempted fate.) Stanley took Len Alyward aside one Saturday morning and said simply: 'We've lost it, the baby.'

'Bad luck, old squire,' Len said, 'but not to worry, there'll be others. Plenty more where that came from, eh?' He punched Stanley playfully on the arm.

Stanley felt a sharp pang of anger. He wanted to catch Len by the throat and throttle him. The idea of the child was festering inside him, poisoning him.

'She's not robust, you know,' he said evenly, 'Irene.'

It was one of her secrets, Stanley knew. Irene had taken great care to give the impression that she had worked at Granitefield but had not been a patient, for fear of being driven out again for being unclean. Len nodded sagely.

Galvanised by a rush of malice, Stanley went on.

'She may never go full term.' There, he thought spitefully, but it wasn't enough. 'It's the TB, you see, it's left a weakness.' Tellingly, he tapped his temple.

Antarctica

MARY O'DONNELL

I do not know what other women know.
I covet their children; wardrobes
stocked with blue or pink, froth-lace
bootees for the animal-child
that bleeds them.

Their calmness settles like the
ebb-tide on island shores—
nursing pearl-conch, secret fronds
of wisdom, certitude.
Their bellies taunt.

I do not know what other women know.
Breasts await the animal-child.
I want—maddened by
lunar crumblings, the false prophecy
of tingling breasts, turgid abdomen.

Antarctica: The storm petrel hovers;
waters petrified by spittled winds:
Little fish will not swim here.
Folds of bed-sheet take my face.
Blood seeps, again.

'But you are free,' they cry,
'You have no child!'—bitterness
from women grafted like young willows,
forced before time. In Antarctica,
who will share this freedom?

Extract from The Light-Makers

MARY O'DONNELL

*This section of the novel is part of the seam of betrayals—
perceived and imagined—which the protagonist Hanna Troy
confronts, in this case when her friend Anna is pregnant. Her
feelings range from outright malice (towards her friend) to some
kind of recognition of the paradoxes involved in birth and
death.*

We are mellow, neither tired nor randy when we go to bed. Sam
sits down, and yanks off his socks, green ones that he wondered
about wearing earlier, thinking they might be too bright. Every
so often he stops and stares at the opposite wall. I undress quickly.
Neither of us will make overtures. In the bathroom I remove
make-up, wash my teeth, pick absently at some congealed soap
in the soap-dish. After washing my face I hold the towel close.
Deeply puzzled. Confused. I wish Kate was here. But there's no
point phoning at this hour. What can I say that would make
sense?

As I stomp back into the bedroom, Sam jerks his head quizzi-
cally. I mumble something about hurrying up. He doesn't re-
ply. I am mortally offended, indignant. So is he but he can't
admit it. We hurt because Anna is pregnant and I am not; we
are galled by it, as if someone viciously lashed at an open wound
and doused it with acid.

'Sam,' I say, not looking at him. He doesn't turn away. What
is it about me that this man refuses to talk? Do I hound him?
Must he retreat into caves of silence every time?

'What?' he says eventually, as if I've just asked the time.

'I can't do any more.'

'I know that. It's all right,' he says softly.

'That's not what I meant!'

He uses this tactic every single time. I throw myself on the
bed. We took trouble with this bedroom. It is warm and com-

forting, as a bedroom should be. The walls are rag-painted in pale green, the paintwork is white and the floor varnished wood with green and yellow Berber rugs. It is the place where the best part of our lives could be lived if only we could get on with it.

'Sam. Please, please see someone!'

'Don't talk nonsense,' he snaps, leaving the room. You'd swear I had asked him to stand on his head naked in the middle of rush-hour traffic.

'You must!' I call, struggling to keep my temper. The bathroom door opens abruptly and he comes back in.

'There's only so much that can be done. Keep taking the tablets for another while.'

'That's just typical of you! Typical of your whole family! None of you can bear the slightest thought of physical imperfection; you have to throw the blame on somebody else!'

He ignores me. I begin to scream. 'Selfish pig! Let me keep taking pills for no bloody reason! They've found nothing bloody wrong with me!' I swipe a book off the floor and leave for the other bedroom.

It is not too much to ask that he has the test done. Or that I become pregnant like many other women my age. Time is running out. It's not as if he has scruples about wanking into a glass tube. He is not hung-up on antediluvian superstitions. But time spills away from us. Every minute lost like sand on the wind. I think back to my childhood, rake the ground of the past for some sign of what was to come. He is so blind that he does not even consider the possible side-effects of those tablets. Twins, triplets, quads and quins. Well stuff it for a business, I don't want multiples.

In biological terms I am old. In a primitive culture I would be a grandmother and I would be respected. I care about being respected. Women envy me; the housebound, those imprisoned by their children. But they also cast me out from among them. Bitter matrons. Men suspect me: barren, witch-woman, seductress. If I don't have children, that must mean I am a selfish, self-seeking, career-oriented bitch who is interested in one thing only.

It is not too much to ask. I am competent. I have passed exams all my life and succeed in almost everything I undertake. Sometimes I dream of a baby. It is soft and naked. I hold it to my bare skin. I have never held a child like that but I am sure of how it feels. There is nothing more delicious, more absolving, more hopeful than the skin of a baby. Such are my dreams.

The bedside light clicks off in the next room. A wind has blown up outside, making a strange moaning sound as it strikes the telegraph wires. What Kate used to call *sí-ghaoth* or fairy-music when Rose and I were children.

We face death. Not having a child forces Sam and me to look at it, eye to eye. We do not always like what we see; there is nothing between us and it. No buffer. No triviality. No light.

Extract from Are You Somebody?

NUALA O'FAOLÁIN

The time and the culture I grew up in proposed to me that somewhere in the creation there was another person—my other half—walking towards me. That person would catch sight of me. But a woman, past the age where she might be contemplated as a sexual partner, is hardly seen. She turns into a silhouette. Nobody scrutinises her detail. She could become a 'character'—in Ireland, anyway. But being avidly watched, because you might at any minute make everyone laugh, is a parody of being watched because you are desired. I met two old ladies in a train in California, on the first leg of a long journey. They were on a frank, not to say raucous, quest for husbands. In Ireland you're not meant to mention love, after a certain age. Yet life teaches you to value love more and more. Human love, if you can secure it. And if you can't, you must hope that other loves will bring you through to the end—for a house or a garden, or a country, or a job increasingly well done, or money, or animals . . . But how can you confer on those the status that loving a person has?

The dog makes me tender. She couldn't believe her luck that Christmas Day. She'd run up the path ahead of me, and then turn and crouch, looking up at my face in her mild and hopeful way, checking that we were still committed to this heavenly activity. We went along behind Newtown Castle, under the flank of the hill, and then we climbed with the little road up to the ridge where there's an old fort and we sat among stones glittering with ice and had our picnic. That night, I would look around the room of the cottage—Molly deeply asleep on her back, her legs sticking straight up, her pink tummy offered to the air—Hodge, the cat, staring, immobile, at the flame of the Christmas candle. I love these animals much more than I want to say. But they are not children.

Rob has a child. He rang me from time to time over the years, usually when someone we'd both known had died. 'I couldn't go to the funeral because I was picking my boy up from school,' he might say, or 'I last saw him when I was taking my boy for a spin on the bike.' One day last year when I was in London he asked me to lunch. I wanted to see him again while I still had my own teeth. So I went to his house and chatted in the big family kitchen with him while he got things ready, and then some friends came and he opened bottles of wine, and then his wife came home from her office and was warmly welcoming to everyone and eventually, nobody wanted to go back to work. Then he and his wife bowed their heads to each other in a quick murmur about domestic arrangements. Then she disappeared for a while. I saw that Rob was watching the door. Then—it was as if the density of the air in the room had changed. A small fair-haired boy in a scuffed school uniform hung in the doorway. He lifted his face to his father in the hope that he wouldn't have to say hello to all of us. This person, waiting to be released to run up to the television, was of a different order from us adults around the table. His head, his soft hair, the school tie badly knotted around his thin neck—the more you looked at him, the more you saw why his father would want to mention him in every sentence—would want to say 'My boy, my boy.' He told us— in a whisper, but confident—that Arsenal would win the Cup. Then his father gave him the nod and he slipped away.

I would have been a very bad mother, during most of my life. But I'd be a good mother, now. Too late. Sometimes I have to look away from small children—hopping where they stand as their mothers try to put on their little jumpers, or talking to themselves pressed against the window in the seat in front of me in the bus. They are too beautiful to bear.

The Authors

Eavan Boland is one of Ireland's leading poets. Her books include *Collected Poems* and *Object Lessons*, a prose collection.

Rory Brennan has worked in education, broadcasting and arts administration. He has lived for long periods in Morocco and Greece. *The Old in Rapallo* is his third collection of verse. He is married with two grown-up daughters.

Mairéad Carew is an archaeologist, currently writing and researching a book entitled 'Tara and the Ark of the Covenant' for the Discovery Programme. She compiled a documentary on cot death, 'Angels in Heaven', for RTE which was broadcast in 1997. In 1993 she won a Listowel Writers' Week Award (short story) and was short-listed for a Hennessy Award (short story) in 1994.

Evelyn Conlon is a novelist, short story writer and mother of two. Her publications include: *My Head is Opening, Stars in the Daytime, Taking Scarlet as a Real Colour* and a forthcoming novel, *A Glassful of Letters*, Blackstaff Press.

Roz Cowman was born in Cork in 1942. She teaches literature and women's studies at University College Cork and elsewhere. Her collection of poems, *The Gooseherd*, was published by Salmon Publishing in 1990.

Peter Cunningham grew up in Waterford. He has been a full-time writer since 1987. His new novel *Consequences of the Heart* will be published in 1998 by The Harvill Press, London.

John F Deane is Director of the Dedalus Press, publishers of new poetry by Irish writers.

Séamus Deane is Keough Professor of Irish Studies, University of Notre Dame. *Reading in the Dark* (1996) won the 1997 Irish Times International Fiction and Irish Fiction Prizes.

Alison Dye grew up in America and moved to Dublin in 1987. In 1989 she won the Stand International Short Story Competition, and in 1994 her first novel, *The Sense of Things*, was shortlisted for the Whitbread First Novel Award. Her second novel, *Memories of Snow*, was published in 1995, followed by *An Awareness of March* in April 1997.

Peter Fallon's books of poems include *The News and Weather* (1987), *Eye to Eye* (1992) and *News of the World: Selected Poems* (1993). He lives in Loughcrew, Co. Meath, where he directs The Gallery Press.

Eleanor Flegg was born in Dublin in 1967 and currently lives in Fife, Scotland. She is married to Christopher Eccles and has two children, Vanya and Turlough. She won a Hennessy Award for her short story 'Daniel in Babylon'.

Hugo Hamilton's latest novel is *Headbanger*, published by Secker and Warburg.

Davoren Hanna was born in Dublin in 1975. Profoundly physically handicapped, he began communicating at the age of seven using a letter board, and later wrote poetry which won awards in Britain and Ireland. Davoren died in 1994.

Kerry Hardie was born in 1951. She was joint winner of a Hennessy Award, winner of Friends Provident/National Poetry Prize 1996, twice winner of the Women's National Poetry Competition and among the prizewinners in Poetry Business, Peterloo, Manchester, Observer/Arvon, Royal Liver, Cardiff International and Staple Open competitions. Her pamphlet, 'In Sickness' was published by *The Honest Ulsterman*.

Michael Hartnett was born in Co. Limerick in 1942. His latest publications include *The Killing of Dreams* (1992) and *Selected and New Poems* (1995).

Seamus Heaney is from Derry and now lives in Dublin. Widely regarded as Ireland's finest living poet, he won the Nobel Prize for Literature in 1995. His *Translation Laments by Jan Kochanowski 1530–1584* with Stanislaw Batranczak was published by Faber in 1996.

Maeve Kelly lives near Limerick. Her most recent works are a collection of short stories *Orange Houses* (1990) and *Alice in Thunderland* (feminist fairy tale) (1993).

Winifred Letts was born in 1882 and died in 1972. Her collection of poems *Songs of Leinster* was published in London in 1913.

Alf McCreary is an author, broadcaster and award-winning journalist who lives and works in Belfast. His most recent book, *An Ordinary Hero*, is a biography of the late Senator Gordon Wilson.

Patsy McGarry, who was born in Ballaghdereen, Co. Roscommon, is the Religious Affairs Correspondent for *The Irish Times*.

Catherine Phil MacCarthy grew up in Co. Limerick. Her poetry collections include *This Hour of the Tide*, Salmon Publishing Ltd (1994) and *The Blue Globe*, due from Blackstaff Press early next year. She was awarded an Arts Council Bursary in 1994, and was Writer in Residence for the City of Dublin, also in that year.

John MacKenna was born in Castledermot, Co. Kildare. His recent publications include *The Fallen* (stories), *Clare* (a novel), *A Year of Our Lives* (stories). *The Last Fine Summer* will be published shortly.

Deirdre Madden is from Co. Antrim. She has published five novels, including *The Birds of the Innocent Wood*, *Nothing is Black*, and *One by One in the Darkness*.

Paula Meehan's most recent book of poems is *Pillow Talk*, published by The Gallery Press. She lives and works in Dublin.

Kuno Meyer was Professor of Celtic in the University of Berlin. He founded the School of Irish Learning in Dublin in 1903.

Mary Morrissy was born in Dublin in 1957. Her first book, a collection of short stories, *A Lazy Eye*, was published in 1993. *Mother of Pearl*, her first novel, won the Lannan Award for literature in 1995 and was shortlisted for the Whitbread Award. She is currently working on her second novel.

Bairbre Ní Chaoimh is a Dublin-based actress and director. She has never written for the theatre before but was inspired to do so by the true story of a woman's search for her natural mother. Together with Yvonne Quinn she researched and co-wrote 'Stolen Child', a full-length play.

Nuala Ní Dhomhnaill has published three books in Irish and three dual-language books. Her forthcoming collection is *Cead Aighnis* (1998).

Eilís Ní Dhuibhne has written several works of fiction, and, under the pseudonym Elizabeth O'Hara, books for children. Her most recent book is *The Inland Ice*, Blackstaff Press.

Máirtín Ó Cadhain (1906–1970), Professor of Modern Irish at Trinity College Dublin, was a teacher and writer of genius. His masterpiece is the novel *Cré na Cille*.

Mary O'Donnell is a poet, novelist, critic and translator. Her publications include *Spiderwoman's Third Avenue Rhapsody* (poetry) and the novels *The Light-Makers* (Poolbeg 1992) and *Virgin and the Boy* (Poolbeg 1996). A collection of stories, *Strong Pagans*, was published in 1991 and many of her stories have subsequently been anthologised. A third collection of poems is due next year. She received an Arts Council literary bursary in 1992.

Bernard O'Donoghue was born in Cullen, Co. Cork in 1945. He has lived in England since 1962, where he teaches Medieval English at Wadham College, Oxford. His most recent volume of poems is *Gunpowder* which won the 1995 Whitbread Prize.

Dennis O'Driscoll was born in Thurles, Co. Tipperary, in 1954. He is a widely-published critic and the author of four collections of poetry, the most recent of which is *Quality Time*, Anvil Press, 1997.

Nuala O'Faoláin is on the staff of *The Irish Times*. Her bestselling autobiography *Are You Somebody?* was published in 1996.

Sheila O'Hagan holds the Patrick Kavanagh Award for Poetry (1991) and the Sunday Tribune/Hennessy Award for New Poet of the Year (1992). Her first collection, *The Peacock's Eye* (1992), was published by Salmon Publishing Ltd, and a second collection, *The Troubled House* followed in February 1995. She has recently completed a writer-in-residency for Kildare County, Ireland.

Cathal Ó Searcaigh grew up in the Donegal Gaeltacht. He is a poet in the Irish language, fast gaining international renown. His work has been translated into French, Italian, German and Catalan.

Derry O'Sullivan was born in Bantry in 1944. He lives in Paris with his wife Jean and three children (Dekin, Isolde, Derval) and teaches at the Sorbonne, ISEP, ICP. His latest collection is *Cá Bhfuil Tiarna Talún L'Univers?* Coiscéim, Dublin.

Siobhán Parkinson is a children's author. *All Shining in the Spring—The Story of a Baby who Died* was shortlisted for the Bisto Award 1995/96. Her teenage novel, *Sisters—No Way!* won the Bisto Award 1996/97. Her most recent novel, for over-tens, is *Four Kids, Three Cats, Two Cows, One Witch (Maybe)*.

Elizabeth Walsh Peavoy was born in December 1945 at Bective, Co. Meath. She is a teacher and media editor. She has three sons. Her daughter Eliza died in Mauritius in 1979 at the age of fourteen months.

Yvonne Quinn was brought up in Dublin but lives in England. She was awarded an Arts Council (England) bursary to develop her writing in 1990. Several of her short stories have been published and two have been broadcast by BBC Radio 4. Her plays include *The Happiness Quotient* (broadcast on RTE).

James Simmons is co-director of the Poets' House, Co. Donegal. His most recent publication is *Elegies*, published by Sotto Voce Press, Maynooth, Co. Kildare. A new collection is forthcoming from Salmon Press.

Janet Shepperson was born in Edinburgh in 1954. She has lived in Belfast since 1977, and has been a creative writing tutor with adult students and in the Maze prison. Her work was included in *The Blackstaff Book of Short Stories* (vols.1&2), and *Trio*, both published by the Blackstaff Press. She has been short-listed twice for a Sunday Tribune/Hennessy Award.

Jason Sommer is a former resident of Howth and tutor at University College Dublin; he now teaches at Fontbonne College, St Louis, Missouri. His poetry has appeared in many magazines, including *The New Republic*, *TriQuarterly*, and *The Honest Ulsterman*. His newest collection, *Other People's Troubles*, has just been published by University of Chicago Press.

INDEX OF AUTHORS